Praise for *Healed through Cancer and Other Adversities*

By James M. Littleton

Healed through Cancer by James Littleton is a treasure trove of faith, scripture quotes, and brotherly advice, as well as a personal account of one man's journey through cancer and the fruits of that journey. With depth and understanding, Littleton takes his readers through the physical, spiritual, and emotional "valley of death" as he learns of his Chronic Lymphocytic Leukemia cancer diagnosis, decides upon and endures various treatments, and wrestles with the issues of living his faith through this experience.

In *Healed through Cancer,* the reader will read moving diary posts that contain wit and wisdom, and consider life's big questions in relationship to suffering, such as the age-old query, "Why ME?" Littleton also addresses the general question that has plagued man from the beginning of time—*why is there suffering in the world and what is its use?*

In *Healed through Cancer,* Littleton:

- shares the four greatest gifts parents can give their children
- offers concrete suggestions for those plagued with worry
- suggests how the role of the sacraments, particularly the sacrament of Confession, aids in total healing
- explains the potent power of prayer using an analogy of donating blood

Imagery is rich and examples are many in this chronicle of faith and fortitude. The author includes an appendix with an examination of conscience and passages of scripture that address healing. Littleton stresses that nothing happens without God's permitting it, and that suffering, when united to Christ's on the Cross, can be redemptive. His story of faith and hope will encourage the cancer stricken, buoy their families, and give faith and light to a suffering world.

—Theresa Thomas,
Today's Catholic News columnist,
author of *Stories for the Homeschool Heart*,
cancer survivor, and
blessed wife and mother of nine

This book is a catechesis for joyful living, written with the eloquence of one who in his sufferings has intimately experienced the love of the Cross. It is for those who suffer from illness, from impatience, from pride, from sin, from fallen human nature...it is a book for everyone. Our Lady of Guadalupe, pray for us.

—David H. Delaney, PhD,
Academic Dean,
Mexican American Catholic College

I am honored to recommend the book *Healed through Cancer*. I was very moved by the author's story depicting his plight in dealing with such an unexpected illness. Having been diagnosed with CLL myself last year, I found the book to be very inspirational for me personally. I truly admire the author for his inner strength, his spirituality, faith, determination, and success in confronting what God has put before him. I urge everyone to read this very inspirational and touching story.

—Maria E. Feldman

In his book, *Healed through Cancer and Other Adversities*, Jim Littleton provides an example of what it means to be a true follower of Christ. When asked by Jesus to "deny himself and take up his cross daily and follow Me" (Luke 9:23), he did just that...and continues to do so. As a Catholic lay evangelist, I constantly stress that our faith involves more than learning facts. Once learned, those facts must also be lived. Here is the story of a man who is doing so in an inspirational and heroic way. I strongly recommend this book for anyone who, like me, tends to lapse into the bad habit of complaining about daily annoyances and who needs a reminder that "God is faithful and will not let you be tried beyond your strength; but with the trial he will also provide a way out, so that you may be able to bear it" (1 Corinthians 10:13)!

—Gary Zimak,
Catholic lay evangelist and radio host

When my wife Kathy and I saw James and Kathleen Littleton on EWTN Live telling the story of *Better by the Dozen, Plus Two*, about their wonderful family of nineteen children (fourteen living), we were impressed.

When, a couple of years later, I received an invitation to review James Littleton's *Healed through Cancer and Other Adversities*, I was delighted. Now that I've finished reading it, I am very much honored and grateful as well.

Healed through Cancer and Other Adversities is a powerful, moving, loving, and very important book. In sharing the story of how he and his family have been impacted by his diagnosis with a particularly aggressive form of Chronic Lymphocytic Leukemia, James Littleton has crafted a book full of joyful, charitable lessons for us all. Far from a sorrowful tome, this book pulls no punches in recounting suffering, but explains with care, wisdom, and humor how it is all worthwhile.

Healed through Cancer and Other Adversities is also a paean of gratitude to God for marriage, parenthood, family life, and all of our abundant blessings. It is a courageous testimony to all human life. You will read, for example, how the author, due to his unyielding respect and love of life, refused to participate in two experimental treatment methods that would have required the use of artificial birth control methods.

Healed through Cancer and Other Adversities is a bountiful resource for those who would understand the meaning of suffering and illness as explained in the scriptures and the teachings of the Catholic Church. Note well the *through* in the title. James shows how God can use even *cancer* as *a means of spiritual healing*. Far from embracing victimhood, Littleton provides hope for the ill and encourages the afflicted themselves to continue to be "pourers," pouring out their love and encouragement to others. I recommend this book without reservation to anyone suffering from cancer or any serious illness or trial, to their family and friends, and to any reader who would care to profit from the heartfelt wisdom and joy of a man who has been blessed with so many good things, and with difficult things as well.

—Kevin Vost, PsyD,
author of *Memorize the Faith!*
and *Three Irish Saints*

God's infinite mercy is for all of us! Author James M. Littleton's faith testimony about the intercession of our Lord Jesus Christ in his life stays strong while he embraces the Cross of cancer, trusting on the miraculous action of the Holy Trinity. The Holy Eucharist and Virgin Mary's Holy Rosary are essential for the spiritual battle. If you are searching for an inspirational spiritual conversion journey experience: *Healed through Cancer and other Adversities* is the book!

—Eduardo Ramos Olivera,
Catholic Screenwriter & Writer

I thoroughly enjoyed and loved reading this book. It will prove to be a source of inspiration to each and every reader. It doesn't matter whether that person has been in the same situation as James Littleton or not. It doesn't matter what the form of sickness, but the truth is this book will provide a wonderful healing spiritually, and also provide a good frame of positive mental attitude, which I believe is so important when one is suffering from ill health.

—Vijay Devadas

What is or has been the length of your mountain range in carrying your cross during your crisis? Be mentored in mind and heart Jim's sacred journey in his love for God and scriptures, and receive miracles of hope! Heaven Offering Perpetual Exhilaration!

—Karen Fulte,
Executive Director,
Bishop Fulton Sheen Spiritual
Centre's Illinois Museum

I found *Healed through Cancer and Other Adversities* inspiring. It will provide hope to many people! It is a healing gratitude book. Many blessings!

—Michael J. Gonzalez Guzman,
Professor at University of Puerto Rico
Medical Sciences Campus

"Everyone in the crowd sought to touch him because power came forth from him and healed them all." (Luke 6:19)

HEALED THROUGH CANCER AND OTHER ADVERSITIES

HEALED
THROUGH
CNCER
AND
OTHER
ADVERSITIES

JAMES M. LITTLETON

Foreword by
Ambassador Michael Novak,
author, philosopher and theologian of liberty,
awarded the Templeton Prize for Progress in Religion in 1994

TATE PUBLISHING
AND ENTERPRISES, LLC

Published by Tate Publishing & Enterprises, LLC
127 E. Trade Center Terrace | Mustang, Oklahoma 73064 USA
1.888.361.9473 | www.tatepublishing.com

Tate Publishing is committed to excellence in the publishing industry. The company reflects the philosophy established by the founders, based on Psalm 68:11,
"The Lord gave the word and great was the company of those who published it."

Book design copyright © 2012 by Tate Publishing, LLC. All rights reserved.
Cover design by Rodrigo Adolfo
Interior design by Caypeeline Casas

Published in the United States of America

ISBN: 978-1-62295-265-6
1. Biography & Autobiography / Medical
2. Religion / Christian Life / Inspirational
12.10.10

Abbreviations and Permissions

DEDICATION

This book is, first and foremost, dedicated to Our Lady of Guadalupe, Mary, the Mother of God, to whom I owe my temporal and eternal life. I also dedicate this book to Venerable Archbishop Fulton J. Sheen, my mentor in heaven, from whom I learned most of what I know about God, philosophy, theology, and the Catholic faith, as well as to Servant of God Archbishop Luis Martinez, another mentor in heaven, from whom I learned much of what I know about the spiritual life. All of the above were my inspirations for writing this book.

ACKNOWLEDGMENTS

How can I convey my love and gratefulness to my inspiration: Kathleen, the love of my life, my bride, the wonderful mother of our nineteen children, an amazing, self-pouring giver, and to each of my children in whose faces I see the Face of God?

I express my gratitude to my eldest daughter, Shannon, who helped tremendously with the editing work, and to my daughter Bridget and J.B. Kelly for their proofing work. I am also grateful to my daughters Fiona, age fifteen; Maura, age fourteen; and Clare, age fourteen, for their extensive help in transcribing dictation for this book. I am grateful to all of my children on earth and in heaven for their support, inspirations, prayers, and prophesies. I express my earnest appreciation to the many munificent, heartening reviewers of this manuscript.

I thank all of the wonderful, generous priests who have touched my life including my spiritual directors over time, Fr. André LaSana, LC, Fr. Colum Power, and Fr. Kevin Baldwin, LC; our parish pastor, Fr. Greg Skowron, and my regular confessor, Fr. Ildephonse Skorup, OFM. I extend a big thank you for the indispensable theological advice provided so generously by Rev. Msgr. Richard Soseman, Congregation for the Clergy, Vatican City. If it were not for our priests we would not have access to the Eucharist and other Sacraments, which strengthen and sanctify us on our earthly pilgrimage toward our heavenly reward.

I extend my inexpressible gratitude to the currently anonymous stem-cell donor who gave me another chance at life.

Thank You, God! Thank you, family! Thank you, everyone!

TABLE OF CONTENTS

FOREWORD

I first met Jim Littleton through his daughter Bridget, a truly talented and accomplished student of mine at Ave Maria University. When he brought up, I asked to see his manuscript on suffering through a possibly fatal cancer, this father of fourteen living, thriving children. If you want to read a beautifully simple and candid book, a spiritually deep book, by a man enduring a particularly lethal cancer, here is your chance.

This brief book that is permeated by a deep Catholic faith, which informs every one of its sentences. It is in Christ's sense childlike and direct. If you have never encountered such an adventure, this is an easily accessible and non-threatening record of human experience too precious to miss.

Ambassador Michael Novak, author, philosopher and theologian of liberty, awarded the *Templeton Prize for Progress in Religion* in 1994[1]

INTRODUCTION

Healed through Cancer and Other Adversities is a profound but deeply personal story of one man's response to serious illness. James Littleton writes of his own story: how a businessman and father of nineteen children, struck by cancer in the form of Chronic Lymphocytic Leukemia, responds to the challenges of such a terrible illness, with the help of his family. He writes of being sustained constantly by their prayers, and by their sacrifices as they ease his discomfort and support one another. Each word of this book is emotionally personal and moving, and manifests the true motivation behind Mr. Littleton's ability to persevere: his faith, which is also the cornerstone of his recovery.

The book consists of a series of meditations, interspersed with a chronology of suffering, treatment, and recovery. Anyone who is suffering from a life-threatening illness, or supporting a family member or friend who so suffers, will find sources of support for their own struggles in the examples found in the book. Anyone who has ever wrestled with life's problems will find resonance with Mr. Littleton's words of his own tremendous challenges.

Healed through Cancer and Other Adversities is certainly a testament to Mr. Littleton's Catholic faith and to the strength and support which this faith offers. The book is, at the same time, eminently accessible and understandable to people of all faiths, or anyone seeking to understand the comforts of faith. Mr. Littleton translates his deeply personal and profound spiritual struggles and thoughts into a style that is pleasing and easy to understand.

Rev. Msgr. Richard Soseman, Vatican City

PROLOGUE

"Blessed be the God and Father of our Lord Jesus Christ, the Father of compassion and God of all encouragement, who encourages us in our every affliction, so that we may be able to encourage those who are in any affliction with the encouragement with which we ourselves are encouraged by God. For as Christ's sufferings overflow to us, so through Christ does our encouragement also overflow" (2 Corinthians 1:3–5).

As I write this I am in the course of treatment for advanced Chronic Lymphocytic Leukemia. I also have the rare 17p chromosome deletion which makes my form of CLL most aggressive and difficult to treat. I am fifty-three years old. I have been happily married for twenty-eight years and have nineteen children: fourteen living, ages five to twenty-five, and five in heaven. I was diagnosed on October 19, 2009. Like St. Paul, in a way, through the course of my life I have experienced "numerous brushes with death" (2 Corinthians 11:23); but unlike St. Paul they mostly happened through my own foolhardiness.

Since my diagnosis I have been facing the possibility of death due to my illness, and I am still facing a questionable prognosis. Nevertheless, God is the Author of Life, and He has preserved my life up until this moment, and until any moment in the future that He decides according to His most perfect and benevolent plan. He seems to have had a mission in mind for me, through which fruit would be borne for others and for His glory. I am exceedingly grateful to Him for this beautiful gift of life.

"Simply reverence the Lord Christ in your hearts, and always have your reason ready for people who ask you the reason for the hope you all have" (1 Peter 3:15–16, JB). I am moved to write this book, *Healed through Cancer and other Adversities*, in an effort to offer hope, encouragement, and fortitude to those carrying the heavy cross of cancer as well as to those carrying the cross in one of its innumerable other forms, and to their loved ones. I want to share my conviction of the unquestionable reality that there is a God, that He cares for each of us personally as if we were the only person He ever created, and that He is bringing a tremendous good out of everything in our lives, especially our crosses—*yes, even cancer!* God is our Merciful Father. He loves each of us infinitely as if he or she were the only person ever created. "Though the mountains leave their place/ and the hills be shaken,/ My love shall never leave you/ nor my covenant of peace be shaken,/ says the LORD, who has mercy on you" (Isaiah 54:10).

I co-authored with my wife, Kathleen, a previous book, published in 2007, *Better by the Dozen, Plus Two: Anecdotes and a Philosophy of Life from a Family of Sixteen*, when I was, or thought I was, in good health—though I suspect this disease may have been with me for years prior to diagnosis. We wrote about the cross, but little did we know that a new cross was in store for us in a few years.

I had procrastinated writing a second book for a bit, but God put it in my heart to get moving. I received encouragement from others including Kathleen. I had been accumulating some random notes with ideas, but I had not gotten down to the hard work of writing in a systematic way. Then in August 2010 Kathleen and I were at Northwestern Hospital in the waiting area prior to my treatment when a man approached us. He commented on the St. Benedict Crucifix and the pin of Our Lady of Guadalupe (Mary, Mother of God) I was wearing and on the fact that I was praying the Liturgy of the Hours. There is a great practical advantage of wearing outward signs of faith, as they open doors to conversations with strangers. It turned out this was Fr. Michael, a Dominican priest. After we had a pleasant conversation, I gave him my business card. He called me the next day sharing that he was moved to call. Knowing that I had previously written a book, he said that I should write a book about my experience with cancer, giving hope and fortitude to others. He had hit on exactly what I was already planning but had been dragging my feet on.

Sometimes God needs to give us a little kick to get us going with the mission to complete His plan of love for which He is counting on us. I took this as a prompting from God to get started. Fr. Michael said that he would be praying and fasting for me. It is interesting that I received a flood of inspirations for this book the next day, which I attribute to Fr. Michael's intercession.

I am a practicing Catholic. I have written this book from a Catholic perspective, which permeates everything for me, although the intended audience is all people of good will—no, I take it back—for people currently of bad will too. After all, the beauty and truth of the Catholic faith are for the benefit of everyone. The reader should know that although I incorporate much Scripture, and comment on theological matters, I am not a formally educated theologian; as a matter of fact, I am not formally educated past high school. But I can read and I can pray, and I have been devouring books, recordings, and other material on the Catholic faith, as well as meditating on the Bible virtually daily for the last twenty years. I can still remember vividly when I first become a religious education teacher at our parish in 1992; I believe it was when I was in a training group. We were asked to bring our Bibles along. The Bible was completely foreign to me at that time. The leader asked that we open to a particular book in the Bible; I think it was to one of the gospels. Well, I looked at this thick book in front of me embarrassed that I had no idea where the passage was to be found. I looked around nervously to see where in the Bible the others were opening to so I could hopefully find my place.

Since my reversion to the Catholic faith in 1991, the Holy Spirit and many spiritual giants such as Venerable Archbishop Fulton J. Sheen, Servant of God Archbishop Luis Martinez, St. John of the Cross, St. Thérèse the Little Flower, St. Faustina Kowalska, Blessed John Paul II the Great, etc. have been my teachers through their writings and recordings, when they were already basking in the presence of God in heaven. How good of a pupil I have been is left to the reader's judgment. A side point: if I can learn my faith and something about Scripture, anyone can.

The reader will notice much repetition where I write about God. True—God is infinite and a mystery beyond even our faintest understanding. Yet there is a dichotomy in this fact that this infinite God and His attributes are profoundly simple, such as love, truth, beauty, and goodness (He is the source of all that is good). Jesus is "the Truth" (John 14:6), and truth has a simplicity about it. Only lies are complicated. So the reader will read much repetition, including about the infinite mercy of God, how He is constantly at work healing us in ways we cannot count, how He loves us beyond our imagination, how He is with us every step of the way, how He is interested in and in command of every detail of our individual lives, about the mystery of how nothing can ever happen outside of His will despite His never interfering with the gift He has given us of free will, about how we are called to have hope and trust in God and to receive His peace, about the value of redemptive suffering, and about how He is bringing a tremendous good out of everything that we encounter in our lives. I cannot avoid repeating these beautiful things as they apply continuously to the themes I have been given the privilege to write about.

Am I writing from the position of self-righteousness? Please God, no! To paraphrase a comment from Venerable Archbishop Fulton J. Sheen, my mentor in heaven, there are many people in jail today, and there is one big difference between them and me—

they got caught; I didn't![2] I have made quite a career as a sinner, though God's grace and infinite mercy have come to the rescue and continue to come to the rescue. I am not the teacher and you the pupil. God forbid! I struggle to live the virtues, truth, and life discussed in this book, and I often fail. But, that makes them no less true, because they are divine. I am not! "Glory to God in the highest" (Luke 2:14, JB), not to me in the lowest. "I am not fit to undo his sandal" (Acts 13:25, JB).

God works His wonders through the most unlikely earthenware jars. "We are only the earthenware jars that hold this treasure, to make it clear that such an overwhelming power comes from God and not from us" (2 Corinthians 4:7–8, JB). I think God often awakens and quickens inspirations and truths that are already hidden in our hearts.

Why the title *Healed through Cancer and other Adversities*? Are cancer and other adversities crosses or transforming, efficacious gifts or both? Well, you will need to read on to get a fuller understanding of the answer to this question. One cannot understand this book without the help of the Holy Spirit. He wants to help us. He has so much truth to say to us because He loves us. "I still have many things to say to you but they would be too much for you now. But when the Spirit of truth comes he will lead you to the complete truth" (John 16:12–13, JB). Approached with reason alone, what I have to say will seem like madness.

I suggest that you pray the following prayer or something similar in your own words:

Come, Holy Spirit, and help me to experience this little book in a state of prayer with the help of your Presence. You are the Father of the Poor, and I am indeed poor and needy in every way. Help me to understand and accept what You wish to reveal to me in this book with great confidence that You always work for my good. Please give me your supernatural understanding and insights. Please give me the fortitude to carry out any changes You want of me, so that I can be happy and at peace, and bring your peace to others. I know You love me infinitely. Please lead me to healing, peace, and joy in every dimension of my life, these gifts which are the fruit of, and mingled with, my painful cross united to yours. I need your help because I am very little and afraid. I trust that You will help and console me whenever I call on you. I invite You as the Sweet Guest of My Soul. I make this prayer with complete confidence in the name of the Father, and of the Son, and of the Holy Spirit. Amen.

Then read this book slowly, not because what I have written is worthy, but because the gentle rain of the Holy Spirit takes a while to soak in. We cannot understand God's ways with reason alone. "And scarce do we guess the things on earth,/ and what is within our grasp we find with difficulty;/ but when things are in heaven, who can search them out?/ Or who ever knew your counsel, except you had given Wisdom/ and sent your holy spirit from on high?" (Wisdom 9:16–17). We need a supernatural perfection of this gift of reason, which comes from grace. Accept this gift!

A divine paradox: mysteriously He is with us, though we must search patiently, but confidently, to find Him. "Truly with you God is hidden,/ the God of Israel, the savior!" (Isaiah 45:15).

The reader may ask, *Why so much Scripture?* What is more profound, sublime, incisive, and helpful than the very Word of God? Certainly not my words! "The word of God is something alive and active: it cuts like any double-edged sword but more finely: it can slip through the place where the soul is divided from the spirit, or joints from the marrow: it can judge the secret emotions and thoughts" (Hebrews 4:12–13, JB).

Sometimes my ramblings seem to go a little off topic, but this is where the Holy Spirit took me. At least this is my excuse.

I hope the reader will benefit from these little wanderings of mine. I pray God will work for your benefit through them, as without Him we "can do nothing" (John 15:5, JB).

Please count on the fact that our combined prayers have already been answered. God has countless inimitable blessings and graces in store for you in this little book planned from all eternity for you personally as His beloved and unrepeatable child. May He be praised and thanked at every opportunity for His goodness and mercy.

Never fear! "By his wounds you have been healed" (1 Peter 2:24).

WHY ME? HEAL ME!

My doctor said to me: "I think you have Chronic Lymphocytic Leukemia."

> Then the mother of Zebedee's sons came with her sons to make a request of him, and bowed low; and he said to her, "What is it you want?" She said to him, "Promise that these two sons of mine may sit one at your right hand and the other at your left in your kingdom." "You do not know what you are asking," Jesus answered. "Can you drink the cup that I am going to drink?" They replied, "We can." "Very well," he said "you shall drink my cup, but as for seats at my right hand and my left, these are not mine to grant; they belong to those to whom they have been allotted by my Father."

> Matthew 20:20–23 (JB)

The cup Jesus was referring to is the sharing of His cross, which is, in God's mysterious, but perfect ways, purifying, healing, redemptive, and effective in transforming us into His apostles and in working to bring others to Christ and in giving God glory.

I was one of those men who very rarely went to the doctor, other than to get some antibiotics for an illness. I had enjoyed excellent health my entire life. I had taken this for granted. I was athletic, in good physical condition with a black belt in Kenpo karate. I had run a couple of marathons. I would walk, jog, play basketball, and do calisthenics to keep fit in recent years.

In late October 2009 I visited a new family-practice doctor for the first time. I did not have a regular doctor. I had a chronic hoarseness and night sweats, which I was concerned about. I thought I had a problem with my throat. The doctor found enlarged lymph nodes in my neck and had a comprehensive blood test run. I received a call from her to come back into her office. When I met with her she told me that my white blood cells were very elevated, and she provided a provisional diagnosis of Chronic Lymphocytic Leukemia (CLL), which was later confirmed by a hematologist/oncologist as stage IV CLL. In the following month or so I learned that I also have the rare 17p chromosome deletion that makes my form of CLL most aggressive and difficult to treat.

I learned that my prognosis was not very promising but that there were chemotherapy and immunotherapy treatments that could help; however, it eventually became clear that I would need a stem-cell transplant, also known as a bone-marrow transplant, which was risky in terms of mortality, but which also held out the reasonable hope of a remission or cure.

It was then the moment to turn to the theological virtue of hope. "Hope is the theological virtue by which we desire the kingdom of heaven and eternal life as our happiness, placing our trust in Christ's promises and relying not on our own strength, but on the help of the grace of the Holy Spirit" (CCC 1817).

Hope is such a beautiful virtue, which we must beg for an increase in from our Blessed Lord. It is good to hope for a physical healing from cancer or other serious ailments. Life is beautiful. Every moment is a gem. There are so many opportunities to grow in love in this life, to grow closer to our infinitely loving God. We must trust in God completely. The truth is, nevertheless, that none of us can have our lives indefinitely prolonged. There comes a moment, a perfect moment, in which God will call each of us to Himself. This cannot happen until He says so. God's timing is always perfect. He arranges every moment and circumstance for our good.

The ultimate good is our salvation, to implore God's always-available, infinite mercy, so we can be gifted with heaven and be with God, and be perfectly happy glorifying Him for all eternity. "We know that by turning everything to their good God co-operates with all those who love him, with all those that he has called according to his purpose. They are the ones he chose specially long ago and intended to become true images of his Son" (Romans 8:28–30, JB).

Yes, God turns everything to its good, no exceptions—yes, even our faults, failings, and sins, which humiliate and humble us and tend to make us more forgiving toward others.

Do we believe that God can even bring a tremendous good out of our sins? Pay attention to this! At the Easter Vigil Mass each year a beautiful prayer is prayed which includes the following: "O truly necessary sin of Adam, destroyed completely by the Death of Christ! O happy fault that earned so great, so glorious a Redeemer!" (RM). How can Adam's sin be called happy and necessary? True, Adam's sin offended God and brought many consequences with it; however, had Adam not sinned there would not have been a need for God to become man, as Jesus, to lift us up, sanctify us, yes, and even divinize us. As a result of Adam's sin, Jesus established his Church, which is His living Mystical Body, to give us the Sacraments including Baptism, which makes us each priest, prophet, and king. The graces Jesus brought to us transform us into His very self so that when the Father gazes upon us He sees Jesus. Did Adam have all this before he sinned? No! We now have infinitely more than Adam had before he sinned.

> Adam prefigured the One to come, but the gift itself considerably outweighed the fall. If it is certain that through one man's fall so many died, it is even more

certain that divine grace, coming through the one man, Jesus Christ, came to so many as an abundant free gift. The results of the gift also outweigh the results of one man's sin: for after one single fall came judgement with a verdict of condemnation, now after many falls comes grace with its verdict of acquittal. If it is certain that death reigned over everyone as the consequence of one man's fall, it is even more certain that one man, Jesus Christ, will cause everyone to reign in life who receives the free gift that he does not deserve, of being made righteous. Again, as one man's fall brought condemnation on everyone, so the good act of one man brings everyone life and makes them justified. As by one man's disobedience many were made sinners, so by one man's obedience many will be made righteous. When law came it was to multiply the opportunities of falling, but however great the number of sins committed, grace was even greater; and so, just as sin reigned wherever there was death, so grace will reign to bring eternal life thanks to the righteousness that comes through Jesus Christ Our Lord.

Romans 5:15–21 (JB)

Never despair of God's mercy. "Let us be confident, then, in approaching the throne of grace, that we shall have mercy from him and find grace when we are in need of help" (Hebrews 4:16, JB).

If you want a dim glimpse into how much God loves each of us, no exceptions (we can never completely comprehend the infinity of this love), look at and contemplate a crucifix, with Jesus, God and man, hanging there for us. He did not come to save the righteous but sinners of which I admit I am one in a big way. How about you? May each of us admit and embrace with confidence and certainty that the infinite mercy of Jesus is available to each of us if we only reach out and accept it. Someone once said something to the effect that there are many unclaimed graces hanging from strings from heaven that are only waiting for us to cut the strings. The scissors are prayer.

I am, of course, not saying that we have a license to sin, presumptuous of God's mercy. We should never play God for the fool! We do not want to offend the One we love the most. But we need to have confidence that God does bring a great good even out of our sins. This good may often be hidden to us, but sometimes God gives us a glimpse. In my case, had I not been the sinner that I was, I would not have the credibility and influence that I have in what I write and speak about. Can not most of you relate to me better, the admitted sinner that I am, than if I had been or claimed to have been virtually perfect since the moment of my birth?

Thanks be to Jesus for His awesome mercy. Thank You, Jesus, for pouring Your healing balm into our wounds. Thank You for bringing us Your peace. "Jesus came and stood among them. He said to them, 'Peace be with you', and showed them his hands and his side" (John 20:20, JB).

So it is good to keep things in perspective. It is good to pray for a healing and a prolongation of our lives: "Father, if you are willing, take this cup away from me", but with a caveat of: "still, not my will but yours be done." (Luke 22:42).

And where did this cup of redemptive suffering come from? "Jesus said to Peter…'Shall I not drink the cup that the Father gave me?'" (John 18:11). The cup came from the *Father*. Note the disciples of Jesus praying to the Father: "Indeed they gathered in this city against your holy servant Jesus whom you anointed, Herod and Pontius Pilate, together with the Gentiles and the peoples of Israel, to do what your hand and [your] will had long ago planned to take place" (Acts 4:27–28). See, this cup of suffering was what the Father's hand and will had always planned.

Why this cup? Out of love for us, God gives this cup so that a tremendous good would come from the suffering and death of His only Son, Jesus, that being our eternal salvation. Why me? Why Jesus? The answer is the same—our Father's will for the salvation of souls, our own and others, for His glory.

Why the cross? Why suffering? Why pain? Certainly there is some mystery involved. But we can be sure that the cross is purifying and redemptive both for us and others. The old adage applies: *No pain, no gain.*

The physical order mirrors the truth and reality of the spiritual order. A few examples would include the following. A mother goes through extreme pain in labor only to receive the marvelous gift of a baby. The horrible pain is soon forgotten (well, I suppose to some extent). We exercise to get or stay in shape, suffering fatigue and various pains in order to be rewarded with a healthier body in good condition, and perhaps a prolonged life. A student sacrifices to study and work hard in order to be rewarded with a developed mind and the necessary skills to work efficaciously in society. We sacrifice activity for sleep in order to be refreshed. We make the sacrifice to go to work, often for long hours so that we might provide sustenance for ourselves and our family. We visit the dentist to have a cavity filled, which can be a painful experience, but the end result is healthy teeth and a winning smile.

"It is necessary for us to undergo many hardships to enter the kingdom of God" (Acts 14:22). That kingdom definitely starts here on earth and is not to be put off for even a moment. Entering the kingdom means being part of the Mystical Body of Jesus. This is how we are healed and purified.

It is best to embrace God's will, which is perfect and always working toward our good. What we can be certain about in reference to His will is that the moment we have before us now is beyond doubt encompassed in His will. We must use each moment well, live life to the full joyfully, have mercy on others and on ourselves, love and serve others at every opportunity. God help me to live this better!

Let us be grateful to God for each moment that He gives us. As I said, *each moment is a gem*! We will never pass this way again, this moment of encounter with God, encounter with others, circumstance, redemptive pain, whatever it may be in His magnificent plan! Thank You for everything, Jesus! Help us to live well every moment of this beautiful gift of life You have given us.

Here is another glimpse into the question, "Why me? Why have I experienced this cross?" John 9:1–41 (JB):

> As he went along, he saw a man who had been blind from birth. His disciples asked him, "Rabbi, who sinned, this man or his parents, for him to have been born blind?" "Neither he nor his parents sinned," Jesus answered "he was born blind so that the works of God might be displayed in him. As long as the day lasts I must carry out the work of the one who sent me; the night will soon be here when no one can work. As long as I am in the world I am the light of the world."

So we see that the blindness, the cross that the man had suffered from birth, was not because of his sin or the sins of his parents. It was *so that the works of God might be displayed in him*. We see how Jesus is teaching that a tremendous good comes out of the cross. Had He Himself not embraced the *night to come* when no one can work by dying on the cross for us, and then risen from the dead three days later, we would have no hope of salvation. Our work and effort only have true eternal value and efficacy when done in union with Christ. Jesus reveals Himself as the *light of the world*. We are each called to imitate Him by carrying out the work of our Father according to our own mission and possibilities.

"Having said this, he spat on the ground, made a paste with the spittle, put this over the eyes of the blind man and said to him, 'Go and wash in the Pool of Siloam,' (a name that means 'sent') So the blind man went off and washed himself and came away with his sight restored." Here we see how Jesus uses His Body and the created things of this world as signs and means of conferring His grace. He employs His sublime, perfect Body, even His spittle— as everything about Him was inconceivably holy: His consoling, wonderful voice; His warm, comforting, gentle touch; His infinitely loving gaze, all of which He took on in the Incarnation out of love of us and to confer grace. This action of Jesus points to the seven Sacraments Jesus instituted for His holy Catholic Church, such as the water used in Baptism; holy oils used in Baptism, Confirmation, and Holy Orders (in other words, ordination to the various degrees of the priesthood); the bread and wine used in Holy Mass which are transformed into the true and actual Body, Blood, Soul, and Divinity of Jesus Christ; and the humanity of the priest when he raises his hand and confers absolution in the Sacrament of Penance (Confession), as he acts *in persona Christi* (in the person of Christ).

As human beings, don't we need the assurance of these concrete signs? Many say that they confess their sins to God directly, but there is nothing like the peace and assurance that come when Jesus forgives our sins through the priest acting *in persona Christi,* as the priest raises his hand and we hear the words of absolution:

> God, the Father of mercies, through the death and the resurrection of his Son has reconciled the world to himself and sent the Holy Spirit among us for the forgiveness of sins; through the ministry of the Church may God give you pardon and peace, and I absolve you from your sins in the name of the Father, and of the Son and of the Holy Spirit.[3]

> CCC 1449

What a sublime grace it is to hear these words spoken to us by Jesus through His priest.

For those Catholics who want to prepare well for a good confession, as well as others who would also like to examine their consciences, I have included an *Examination of Conscience* in the appendix. It may be a little difficult to understand, so turn to the Holy Spirit for help in understanding these spiritual and moral realities. Don't be afraid. I am not proud of this, but I have committed most every sin on this list in the course of my life in some shape or form. Confession is the "Sacrament of Mercy." We can take solace in the following scripture: "However great the number of sins committed, grace was even greater" (Romans 5:21, JB). I have also included a *Guide to Confession: How to Go to Confession.*

We also see here the faith that the blind man exercised in following the instruction of Jesus, which would not make much sense on a human level, when he went and washed in the Pool of Siloam. The blind man was sent to this pool called "sent," and once healed would be sent to others to proclaim what the good God had done for Him to help bring them to the gift of faith, and to give God glory.

> His neighbors and people who earlier had seen him begging said, "Isn't this the man who used to sit and beg?" Some said, "Yes, it is the same one." Others said, "No, he only looks like him." The man himself said, "I am the man." So they said to him, "Then how do your eyes come to be open?" "The man called Jesus" he answered "made a paste, daubed my eyes with it and said to me, 'Go and wash at Siloam'; so I went, and when I washed I could see." They asked, "Where is he?" "I don't know." He answered.

Once we begin to be healed and transformed by Jesus it is usually the case that the people around us in our lives will become confused when observing the changes in us, which have come about through no merit of our own, but through the grace of God.

It is sometimes difficult for them to comprehend the invisible at work in us—the things of the Spirit, Who has been poured out upon us. We may not have all the insights and answers, but the change and fruits in us are undeniable.

> They brought the man who had been blind to the Pharisees. It had been a Sabbath day when Jesus made the paste and opened the man's eyes, so when the Pharisees asked him how he had come to see, he said, "He put a paste on my eyes, and I washed, and I can see." Then some of the Pharisees said "This man can not be from God: he does not keep the Sabbath." Others said, "How could a sinner produce signs like this?" And there was disagreement among them. So they spoke to the blind man again, "What have you to say about him yourself now that he has opened your eyes?" "He is a prophet" replied the man.

We see how the blind man is just beginning to comprehend and have faith in Jesus, and to understand Who He is. We can also notice the confusion among the Pharisees, some not believing and being hypercritical, and others beginning to be transformed themselves. *How can a sinner produce fruits like this?* Is this not the experience of the people in our lives when we begin to *live Christ*?

The blind man is beginning to have some experience of St. Paul who said, "Life to me, of course, is Christ" (Philippians 1:21, JB). This man, who has been healed from his blindness, is a figure of how Jesus heals us and brings us into the light of his truth and mercy. He is experiencing a deep transformation that is available to each of us, "and for anyone who is in Christ, there is a new creation; the old creation has gone, and now the new one is here. It is all God's work" (2 Corinthians 5:17–18, JB). He is beginning to experience the sentiments of St. Paul: "The love of Christ overwhelms us" (2 Corinthians 5:14, JB). This healing and transformation that we experience is not due to any merit on our part. *It is all God's work.*

> However, the Jews would not believe that the man was blind and had gained his sight without first sending for his parents and asking them, "Is this man really your son who you say was born blind? If so, how is it that he is able to see?" His parents answered, "We know that he is our son and we know that he was born blind, but we don't know how it is that he can see or who opened his eyes. He is old enough: let him speak for himself." His parents spoke like this out of fear for the Jews who had already agreed to expel from the synagogue any one who should acknowledge Jesus as the Christ. This is why his parents said, "He is old enough; ask him."

We see here a representation of how, once we begin to be transformed by and into Christ, even those family members and friends closest to us are often not ready to understand. They may react out of fear as they contemplate the possible truth and reality of what has happened, while asking themselves what it would cost them to follow Christ. We can be confident, however, that when we fervently pray and sacrifice for them they will, in God's time, be converted and transformed as well, and we will spend eternity most happily in heaven with those we love the most.

> So the Jews again sent for the man and said to him, "Give Glory to God! For our part we know that this man is a sinner." The man answered, "I don't know if he is a sinner; I only know that I was blind and now I can see." They said to him, "What did he do for you? How did he open your eyes?" He replied, "I have told you once and you wouldn't listen. Why do you want to hear it all again? Do you want to become his disciples too?" At this they hurled abuse at

him. "You can be his disciple," they said "We're disciples of Moses: we know that God spoke to Moses, but as for this man we don't know where he comes from." The man replied, "Now here is an astonishing thing! He has opened my eyes and you don't know where he comes from! We know that God doesn't listen to sinners, but God does listen to men who are devout and do his will. Ever since the world began it is unheard of for anyone to open the eyes of a man who was born blind; if this man were not from God, he couldn't do a thing." "Are you trying to teach us," they replied "and you a sinner through and through since you were born!" And they drove him away.

When we begin to live the truth and follow Christ, we can count on abuse and persecution from some. This is an absolute. We must, however, persevere through this. Jesus said, "Alas for you when the world speaks well of you!" (Luke 6:26, JB). We who are beginning to be transformed by Christ are often seen as a threat to those around us by the example of our lives which call them to conversion. They wonder why we are not living the same way as they are, like we used to. Some will not want anything to do with us any longer—*and they drove him away.*

Jesus heard they had driven him away, and when he found him he said to him "Do you believe in the son of man?" "Sir," the man replied "tell me who he is that I may believe in him." Jesus said "You are looking at him; he is speaking to you." The man said "Lord, I believe", and worshipped him.

We see how Jesus did not and would never abandon this man who had been born blind. He sought him out when in trouble. He sought his faith. The man responded well with the words we should all imitate, "Lord, I believe." We should imitate the faith of this man by worshiping Jesus in "spirit and truth" (John 4:24, JB).

"Jesus said: 'It is for judgment that I have come into the world, so that those without sight may see and those with sight may turn blind.'" We see how blindness is a metaphor for being in the dark without our savior, Jesus Christ. When we allow Him into our lives, we come into the light. It is true that in the light we find various forms of the cross, but this is the only way to an elevated height of love and conversion.

We should try to keep in mind that after the cross of Good Friday comes the Resurrection of Easter. Through our crosses, we have been chosen by Christ to help Him redeem the world. What a privilege! The following quote is worth many repetitions in this little book: "It makes me happy to suffer for you, as I am suffering now, and in my own body to do what I can to make up all that has still to be undergone by Christ for the sake of his body, the Church" (Colossians 1:24–25, JB).

May we have the experience of St. Paul as regards the cross:

> During my stay with you, the only knowledge I claimed to have was about Jesus, and only about him as the crucified Christ. Far from relying on any power of my own, I came upon you in great "fear and trembling" and in my speeches and the sermons that I gave, there were none of the arguments that belong to philosophy; only a demonstration of the power of the Spirit. And I did this so your faith should not depend on human philosophy but on the power of God.
>
> 1 Corinthians 2:2–5 (JB)

It is apropos to borrow an insight from Venerable Archbishop Fulton J. Sheen.[4] When St. Paul first went to Corinth he had just left Athens where he had preached at the great Council of the Areopagus. He had had limited success in winning converts to Christianity in Athens, I think because he relied too much on himself, and not on Christ. He spoke in terms of philosophy, in which he was well trained, and skipped right over the crucifixion of Jesus to the resurrection. He learned from this experience so that from then on he preached and lived the cross of Christ. At Corinth Jesus encouraged St. Paul:

> One night the Lord spoke to Paul in a vision, "Do not be afraid to speak out, nor allow yourself to be silenced: I am with you. I have so many people on my side in this city that no one will even attempt to hurt you." So Paul stayed there preaching the word of God among them for eighteen months.

> Acts 18:9–11 (JB)

Returning to John 9:1–41 (JB) we read,

> Jesus said: "It is for judgment that I have come into the world, so that those without sight may see and those with sight may turn blind." Hearing this, some Pharisees who were present said to him, "We are not blind, surely?" Jesus replied: "Blind? If you were you would not be guilty, but since you say, 'We see', your guilt remains."

May we all admit to Jesus that we are blind without Him and seek His always readily available healing and forgiveness.

WHO AM I THAT NEEDS HEALING?

"I and the children whom Yahweh has given me are signs and portents in Israel from Yahweh Sabaoth who dwells on Mount Zion" (Isaiah 8:18, JB).

As I write this portion in March 2011, I am fifty-two years old. I have been married to my wonderful bride, Kathleen, for twenty-seven years. God blessed us with nineteen children through no merit of our own. Our living children, aged twenty-five to five, are: Shannon Rose, Tara Kathleen, Grace Ellen, Colleen Anne, Deirdre Marie, Bridget Jane, Shane Francis, Fiona Mary, Maura Therese, Clare Margaret, Patrick Michael, Mairead Siobhan, Brighde Rosemarie, Shealagh Maeve; and our miscarried and still born children are: Maximilian Mary, Theresa Gerard, James Paul, Frances Xavier, and Joseph Faustina.

I grew up in the middle class in a fine family on the South Side of Chicago. I was raised Catholic but did not practice my faith very well. By the time I reached age thirteen I began to live a very sinful and dissolute life. You could perhaps find me on weekends at 1:00 a.m. walking down Western Avenue with a cigarette dangling from my mouth and a bottle of wine tucked under my coat, drunk as can be. This was not my wonderful parents' fault, by the way. I was entirely uncontrollable.

As I grew, I was a hedonist, totally self-centered, mean, cruel, and getting in all sorts of trouble—most of which I never got caught for.

I was a regular at a local bar at about age sixteen. As a teenager and young man I got drunk practically every night or would at least drink to excess. There were many sins in my life. I certainly broke every commandment. I did not murder anyone, so I thought I was better than I was, although in actual fact I did break the fifth commandment, "You shall not kill" (Exodus 20:13), by endangering myself and others often with my behavior.

I eventually met Kathleen in my early twenties, a miracle of miracles. We were married in 1983. I had no formal education past high school. She was beautiful and was finishing up law school. This was only possible by the grace of God's most perfect providence.

When I had met Kathleen I was at a party at the University of Illinois at Champaign. I was a dock worker at UPS. I had gone to the U of I just for the party as I did not attend the university. I saw Kathleen across the room and experienced an amazing moment of grace where I knew with certainty that we were going to be married. I could not explain this at the time, but I now see this as a movement of the Holy Spirit. I introduced myself to her and told her that she was going to be my bride. This, of course, initially made her think I was crazy. But I pursued her for a couple of years and eventually, by God's grace, won her over, as can now be attested to by the existence of our nineteen children.

To make a long story short, we regrettably started off our marriage contracepting, which is contrary to the Catholic Church's profound teaching regarding openness to life. After a year or two, Kathleen was moved to stop taking the Pill. We quickly conceived our first child, Shannon Rose.

At this point in my life most people would have considered me a good family man, although I was still drinking too much and was a major sinner in numerous ways. Then in 1991 when we had five children, I had a major conversion to the fullness of the Catholic faith. After this conversion I was healed in many ways from my sinfulness, though I still struggle with many faults as my conversion continues. By the grace of God I left the heavy drinking behind many years ago.

My conversion happened when there was a report of the Blessed Virgin Mary appearing in Hillside, a suburb of Chicago, at Queen of Heaven Cemetery. I packed up Kathleen and the kids in the car and went there with the purpose of looking for signs more than any piety on my part. I did not see any provable miracles, though there were some interesting signs. But I was moved powerfully by the Holy Spirit. I was particularly influenced by the striking piety of the people praying there. The Holy Spirit showered tremendous graces on me through no merit of my own. I was being *healed* by God through the intercession of the Blessed Virgin Mary, and I experienced a profound peace and the presence of God.

Someone handed me a holy card of the fifteen promises of Mary to those who pray the rosary. I took this holy card and put it on my dresser where I generally ignored it for about a year. Then one day I decided to start praying the rosary. I could not recall how to pray it, so I believe I went to a local Catholic gift shop where I obtained a rosary and a pamphlet. I began by praying one decade of the rosary per day, in other words, twelve short prayers that take about three minutes to pray. I thought to myself that it was hard to believe that any one could pray so much in one day—three whole minutes!

Soon I was praying the entire rosary each day. In a short time it occurred to me that Mass was probably offered at my parish daily, which of course it was. One morning I went to Mass on a weekday, which is not required of a Catholic like Sunday Mass, though it is highly recommended to attend daily. At this Mass I was once again overwhelmed by an outpouring of the Holy Spirit. I experienced God's love and presence in a deep and powerful way, with tears cascading uncontrollably down my face.

Soon I was going to Mass every day except Saturday, presuming that God would know that I would need to sleep in on Saturdays. That false reasoning quickly fell aside; I began attending Mass on Saturday too. Soon I was moved by the Holy Spirit with an understanding that if attendance at Holy Mass was the greatest thing one could do for himself with infinite graces available for the taking, how could I leave my children at home? So I began to bring all of my children, except the ones in diapers, thereby still falling short of what God wanted me to do. I reasoned that certainly God would understand that I could not be bothered changing babies' diapers at Mass.

About eight years later Kathleen was moved to come to daily Mass with us, and she has never missed a day since except when in the hospital delivering babies. The day the baby came home she resumed daily Mass attendance with us along with the new baby. We have attended daily Mass as a complete family ever since— all of us, from newborn to parents. Those of our children who are away at college and such have continued the practice of daily Mass attendance.

We began to pray daily as a family including the rosary and Scripture. Our family also began to attend the Sacrament of Reconciliation weekly, which has been a tremendous grace for us. We embarked on attending Eucharistic adoration regularly (praying before the Eucharist, truly Jesus's Body, Blood Soul and Divinity, exposed for adoration in the monstrance). This was all God's gift. All glory to Him!

Our children became very active in the Catholic groups in the Church. Kathleen and I engaged in many forms of ministry including spiritual direction for others, by God's grace.

Who am I? I am an imperfect sinner, *whose sins are as scarlet*, but who has been on a powerful road of conversion for the past twenty years. (Why is it taking so long for me to be purified, Lord?) I am exceedingly grateful to God for His inexhaustible patience and mercy toward me. "Though your sins are like scarlet, they shall be as white as snow; though they are red as crimson, they shall be like wool" (Isaiah 1:18, JB). By God's grace, I am now a man who puts God and His things first in my life. Second is my wife, and third is my children. Work comes in fourth place and ministry fifth, though I make room for all of these.

Believe me, if God can lead me, a major sinner, to conversion, he can lead anyone!

> I thank Christ Jesus our Lord, who has given me strength, and who judged me faithful enough to call me into his service even though I used to be a blasphemer and did all I could to injure and discredit the faith. Mercy, however, was shown me, because until I became a believer I had been acting in ignorance; and the grace of our Lord filled me with faith and with the love that is in Christ Jesus. Here is a saying that you can rely on and nobody should doubt: that Christ Jesus came into the world to save sinners. I myself am the greatest of them; and if mercy has been shown to me, it is because Jesus Christ meant to make me the greatest evidence of his inexhaustible patience for all the other people who later have to trust in him to come to eternal life.
>
> 1 Timothy 1:12–17 (JB)

As I am sure would apply to most people with cancer, I never expected to be suffering from leukemia. This is very difficult on a human level; however, I know that it is encompassed in God's will where He is mysteriously bringing a tremendous good out of it for me and for others who I pray and intercede for. Glory to God in the highest! "Glory to God in the highest heaven" (Luke 2:14, JB).

HEALING THROUGH GOD, BUT DOES HE EXIST?

He is the image of the invisible God,/ the firstborn of all creation./ For in him were created all things in heaven and on earth,/ the visible and the invisible,/ whether thrones or dominions or principalities or powers;/ all things were created through him and for him./ He is before all things,/ and in him all things hold together./ He is the head of the body, the church./ He is the beginning, the firstborn from the dead,/ that in all things he himself might be preeminent./ For in him all the fullness was pleased to dwell,/ and through him to reconcile all things for him,/ making peace by the blood of his cross [through him],/ whether those on earth or those in heaven./ And you who once were alienated and hostile in mind because of evil deeds he has now reconciled in his fleshly body through his death, to present you holy, without blemish, and irreproachable before him, provided that you persevere in the faith, firmly grounded, stable, and not shifting from the hope of the gospel that you heard, which has been preached to every creature under heaven, of which I, Paul, am a minister.

Colossians 1:15–23

As a younger man I tended toward believing in God with lip service, though I generally lived and acted as if I did not believe He existed. I most certainly did not have a loving relationship with Him. But, He never gave up on me, as He never gives up on you. I eventually received from His hands the paramount gift of faith, through no merit of my own. This gift is available to every one of us for the asking, though it will never be imposed upon us.

Perhaps the reader is struggling with the question "Does God exist?" The answer is an unequivocal "Yes!" By the way, His existence does not depend upon our acquiescence. He is! How can we sum up Who God is, but in His own words, too deep to fully penetrate with our weak mortal minds: "I Am" (John 8:58, JB). Not "I was," or "I will be," but "I am."

Do you believe in the one true God? If not, then what or who do you believe in? Everyone has a god. What are my gods: my intellect, science, money, possessions, power, prestige, sex, leisure, my stomach, technology, politics, my body? We could go on and on. These are not bad things in themselves when used in an ordered and proper way, when we use them for the good of ourselves and others and the glory of God. The trouble comes when we make gods of something other than the one true God. The false gods we choose ultimately own and enslave us. We surrender our freedom, which is a supreme gift from our true God, and submit to these enslavers. Will these false gods comfort us and give us peace as we take our leave of this world one day, on a day we do not know, but which is certain to come? Have you ever known of anyone taking any of these things into eternity?

The most common god we can naturally tend to choose is ourselves, whether we do so knowingly or not. It is very common for persons today to be moral relativists wherein they choose and create their own moral "truths" to live by, which they claim not to impose on anyone else. They claim to be tolerant of everyone else's right to choose their own set of moral beliefs, but watch out if someone else's beliefs interfere in some way with theirs. In other words they have fooled themselves into believing that they themselves can establish what is right and wrong for themselves while claiming that there is no such thing as objective truth that applies to everyone. Of course, this proclamation that there is no binding, universal, objective truth is ipso facto paradoxically presented as an objective truth in itself that should apply to everyone. And you have committed a terrible mortal sin should you burst their bubble claiming that there is an objective truth that is binding to everyone including them. Theirs is a preposterous philosophy, which virtually all of us have been unduly influenced by, as the culture we live and breathe in is so completely saturated by it.

Those who live as moral relativists may claim that they believe in God, but they believe and live as if they are all powerful and can tell God what is right and wrong, which in fact infers that they are more omnipotent than the God they claim to believe in. God, for them, becomes a puppet of their own will. But this is far from the truth of who the one true God is. God is God. We are not.

Of course we all have the tendency to be personally biased in justifying the things we want to do, even if this hurts others, myself most definitely included. That is why we need God. We need His help in coming to the Truth, understanding it, embracing it, and living it. As a matter of fact, the Truth is not something abstract. The Truth is a Person, Jesus, the second Person of the Most Holy Trinity. We can know the truth and are enabled to live it better when we fall in love with Him—that is to say when we fall in love with the Truth. *We fall in love with Love.*

Jesus tells us: "I am the Way, the Truth and the Life" (John 14:6, JB). Jesus is the only way to the Truth and Life; He is the

Truth; and this Truth, this Jesus, who is the true Life, gives us life eternal. We cannot attain this by ourselves. We must be lifted up to it by Jesus, through His supernatural help, which does not naturally belong to us, but is always readily available to us if we so desire.

Only God can consecrate us in truth. "Consecrate them in the truth; your word is truth" (John 17:17, JB).

The reality is that we are not determiners of truth. Truth is not something we have the power to invent, but an objective reality that we are called to accept and live. This truth does not oppress us, but rather frees us and makes us happy. "The truth will make you free" (John 8:32, JB).

Well, the truth is that there is one true God and He is the Truth. There are objective truths that apply to everyone, too numerous to even begin to spell out here. The best place to find these truths enumerated is in the *Catechism of the Catholic Church*.[5]

For example, an objective truth is that we should never directly and intentionally kill/abort innocent babies in the womb who are unable to defend themselves. These are unrepeatable, unique persons, full of potential, with unique missions on earth, made in God's own image and likeness, and intended to be perfectly happy for all eternity with God.

God is all powerful and has our eternal destiny in His hands, wanting us all to be saved and to come to be with Him in perfect happiness for all eternity. Why would I not want to know Him, love Him, and serve Him?

Can I provide thousands of reasons that point to the existence of God, such as nature—wherein it seems absurd to think that everything is an accident in regard to mankind—the world, and the universe in their astounding beauty, harmonization, and precision? Yes, God exists. Can I give to the reader a personal assent and assurance by citing reasons and arguments for the existence of God? No! We can never come to an unshakable, living, confident, assured faith in God by our reason alone. Our intellect is too weak and limited. We are finite, while God is infinite. I am not saying that we should not apply our reason, but *our reason must be perfected by grace.*

What a profound and liberating thing it is to come to know, love, and serve the one true God! He never imposes Himself. He offers Himself to us as the *Ultimate Gift!* We need only reach out and accept.

We can only come to faith in God, and act on it, through the aid of something supernatural outside of ourselves. We can only come to this faith, which is built on rock, through the gift of grace, through the gift of faith from God's munificent hands.

> "Everyone who comes to me and listens to my words and acts on them—I will show you what he is like. He is like the man who when he built his house dug, and dug deep, and laid the foundations on rock; when the river was in flood it bore down on that house but could not shake it, it was so well built."

Luke 6:47–49, JB

Yes, faith is a gratuitous gift. "For by grace you have been saved through faith, and this is not from you; it is the gift of God" (Ephesians 2:8). We can only receive this gift if we exercise the gift of our free will to accept it.

Therefore, if the reader doubts the existence of God, and in good faith wishes to at least acknowledge that it is possible that God may in fact exist, then I encourage the reader to simply open his heart, mind, and soul and ask God for this special grace of all graces, exercising his free will to receive and accept this sublime gift of faith. I can assure you that if you do this you will be granted the gift of faith either immediately, or eventually in God's perfect timing. Count on this! Praise be to God Most High for His inexpressible gifts and generosity! This aim is kept in my deepest prayers.

When we believe in God it opens the door for us to turn to Him for all we need, and to trust in Him. It is then that we receive the gift of peace, for which we all innately hunger. Only God can give us this genuine peace. Only God can truly heal us in the various dimensions of our person, including physical health, mind, soul, and spirit. "'But I will heal him, and console him, I will comfort him to the full, both him and his afflicted fellows, bringing praise to their lips. Peace, peace to far and near. I will indeed heal him,' says Yahweh" (Isaiah 57:18–19, JB).

God has all the power, and is always using it for our good. He desires to comfort us and to bring us genuine peace. He wants to heal us in every conceivable way. When we turn to our all-powerful God, He will always hear us and answer every prayer for our good—though sometimes, as with any good father, the answer will be "no" for our own good, with His eye on our ultimate and supreme good, that of our eternal salvation. I guess I can bring myself to thank You, Father, for the times You said "no" when I prayed to win the lottery; You know best. Thank You, Father, for Your constant loving concern for us in every detail of our lives.

HEALING
THROUGH POVERTY

"Therefore I tell you, do not worry about your life, what you will eat [or drink], or about your body, what you will wear. Is not life more than food and the body more than clothing? Look at the birds in the sky; they do not sow or reap, they gather nothing into barns, yet your heavenly Father feeds them. Are not you more important than they? Can any of you by worrying add a single moment to your life-span? Why are you anxious about clothes? Learn from the way the wild flowers grow. They do not work or spin. But I tell you that not even Solomon in all his splendor was clothed like one of them. If God so clothes the grass of the field, which grows today and is thrown into the oven tomorrow, will he not much more provide for you, O you of little faith? So do not worry and say, 'What are we to eat?' or 'What are we to drink?' or 'What are we to wear?' All these things the pagans seek. Your heavenly Father knows that you need them all. But seek first the kingdom [of God] and his righteousness, and all these things will be given you besides. Do not worry about tomorrow; tomorrow will take care of itself. Sufficient for a day is its own evil."

Matthew 6:25–34

January 6, 2010: I am in the hospital on IV antibiotics with a blood clot and cellulitis in my left arm, apparently a complication from chemotherapy. It is interesting that the only reason my cellulitis infection was discovered in time was that I was suffering severe constipation from the medication I was taking, and ended up with an impacted bowel. I visited the emergency room to take care of that when I decided to show the doctor the redness on my arm as an afterthought. He said that if I had waited until the following morning I would have been in big trouble. God writes straight with crooked lines. (I ended up hospitalized a second time with this same cellulitis infection on approximately January 31ˢᵗ as it returned after the initial treatment.)

I know that my illness and the complications I am experiencing are life threatening. I have not been able to work at my business for a couple of months. We have very little income coming in. Many bills are due. The ability to keep my family off the streets and in a home appears in serious jeopardy. I received an e-mail from a friend who had sent a previous gift that had helped us to pay our bills and rent. He wrote that he was sending another check in the mail. This type of scenario has been repeated numerous times in the life of my family. Though we have experienced serious financial difficulties including the foreclosure of our home, our beneficent Father in heaven has always provided what we truly needed, though usually at the last moment. This helps us to learn to trust in Him, not in ourselves or in things. He is our All!

Even when we were about to lose our home through foreclosure in 2007, a community of Poor Clare nuns told us that they were praying to God that if we lost our house we would receive a better one. That is exactly what happened. Though we are now renters, we are living in a home in the perfect location we would prefer with parks, town, stores, and recreation all within close waking distance. The house is perfect for our needs.

None of us really own anything here on earth anyway. We are redeemed strangers and sojourners, on our way to the promised land of heaven in eternity, as long as we exercise our free will to follow God's will to love Him and our neighbor the best we can (though we will all fall short), and given we seek the mercy of Jesus. "So then you are no longer strangers and sojourners, but you are fellow citizens with the holy ones and members of the household of God, built upon the foundation of the apostles and prophets, with Christ Jesus himself as the capstone" (Ephesians 2:19–20).

When we are poor in the things of this world such as money, this is not an obstacle to holiness and happiness. As a matter of fact, Jesus highlights an example of a poor widow as a benchmark of generosity and trust that we are all called to emulate. "When he looked up he saw some wealthy people putting their offerings into the treasury and he noticed a poor widow putting in two small coins. He said, 'I tell you truly, this poor widow put in more than all the rest; for those others have all made offerings from their surplus wealth, but she, from her poverty, has offered her whole livelihood'" (Luke 21:1–4). What did she hold on to? Nothing! She gave everything. She trusted God completely. Do you think God would ever let her down? Do you not think that God saw to this poor widow's needs her entire life and ultimately welcomed her into heaven?

There is another type of poverty. We are all weak and lacking everything good on our own. It is only by God's grace that we can be lifted out of this poverty and be enriched with the things of God, which will last through all eternity. When we recognize this poverty in ourselves, one could say that we have a right to the power and mercy of God to heal us, and use us for the good. We turn to Christ and are made rich in the many gifts He wants to shower upon us. In Christ our lives bear more fruit. But if we are full of ourselves and a false sense of self-sufficiency, there is no room for those graces.

> "My grace is enough for you: my power is at its best in weakness." So I shall be very happy to make my weaknesses my special boast so that the power of Christ may stay over me, and that is why I am quite content with my weaknesses and with insults, hardships, persecutions, and the agonies I go through for Christ's sake. For it is when I am weak that I am strong.
>
> 2 Corinthians 12:9–10 (JB)

God loves to use the weak to perform stupendous deeds. The weaker and poorer we are, the more God works through us. Those of us who suffer from cancer or other crosses are blessed with an increased capacity to understand and live this reality.

There are numerous passages in Scripture where God chooses the least likely, most weak individual to fulfill His amazing plans. An example is Gideon, who with only three hundred soldiers routed Midian's vast army as depicted in Judges 6:14–24 (JB).

> At this Yahweh turned to him and said, "Go in the strength now upholding you and I will rescue Israel from the power of Midian. Do I not send you myself?" Gideon answered him, "Forgive me, my Lord, but how can I deliver Israel? My clan, you must know, is the weakest in Manasseh and I am the least important in my family." Yahweh answered him, "I will be with you and you shall crush Midian as though it were a single man."

It is interesting where Gideon received his power. "Gideon went away and prepared a young goat and made unleavened cakes with an ephah of flour." These represent the Holy Eucharist.

"He put the meat into a basket and the broth into a pot then brought it all to him under the terebinth."

The terebinth, where the angel of Yahweh was seated, represents the cross of Christ. "As he came near, the angel of Yahweh said to him, 'Take the meat and unleavened cakes, put them on this rock and pour the broth over them.'"

The rock represents Christ and the broth His blood. "Then the angel of Yahweh reached out the tip of the staff in his hand and touched the meat and unleavened cakes. Fire sprang from the rock and consumed the meat and unleavened cakes and the angel of Yahweh vanished before his eyes." The fire represents the Holy Spirit.

"Then Gideon knew this was the angel of Yahweh, and he said, 'Alas, my Lord Yahweh! I have seen the angel of Yahweh face to face!' Yahweh answered him, 'Peace be with you; have no fear; you will not die'" (Judges 6:14–24, JB).

So Gideon, the least of the weakest clan in Manasseh, receives his strength from what prefigures the Eucharist. This Holy Eucharist is available daily in the Holy Mass for those who are Catholic. For those who are not, I encourage you to consider accepting the gift of becoming Catholic so that you might partake of this heavenly food. When we receive Jesus in the Eucharist we have Everything. We are no longer poor, but rich.

HEALING
THROUGH DARKNESS

Or a man is chastened on his bed by pain/ and unceasing suffering within his frame,/ So that to his appetite food becomes repulsive,/ and his senses reject the choicest nourishment./ His flesh is wasted so that it cannot be seen,/ and his bones, once invisible, appear;/ His soul draws near to the pit,/ his life to the place of the dead./

If then there be for him an angel,/ one out of a thousand, a mediator,/ To show him what is right for him/ and bring the man back to justice,/ He will take pity on him and say,/ "Deliver him from going down to the pit;/ I have found him a ransom."/ Then his flesh shall become soft as a boy's;/ he shall be again as in the days of his youth./ He shall pray and God will favor him;/ he shall see God's face with rejoicing./ He shall sing before men and say,/ "I sinned and did wrong,/ yet he has not punished me accordingly./ He delivered my soul from passing to the pit,/ and I behold the light of life."

Lo, all these things God does,/ twice, or thrice, for a man,/ Bringing back his soul from the pit/ to the light, in the land of the living.

Job 33:19–30

On November 1, 2009, All Saints' Day, I was hospitalized at St. James Hospital with double pneumonia in my lower lungs. This was only thirteen days following my diagnosis of Chronic Lymphocytic Leukemia. It was extremely painful and difficult to breathe. This was a life-threatening situation.

When one is this sick it affects body, mind, soul, and spirit. I began having fears, anxiety, and experiencing demonic dreams and images. I am so helpless by myself.

I nearly died. I may have died physically for a time. I experienced horrible darkness, demonic attacks, and the heavy weight of my sins. Seeing myself in God's light is so painful. How lax I have been in conscience. How many opportunities I missed in my life to do good. I felt totally alone. I had no sense of the presence of God, though I had faith and hope that He is with me always, loves me, and is infinitely merciful.

Within about ten days I was sufficiently recovered, just a day or so before I left to travel to Alabama with Kathleen for a couple of appearances on the Eternal Word Television Network. Kathleen was very sick too. She was well enough to travel the day we left. We decided to go forward with these television appearances in spite of our illnesses and my personal spiritual darkness, as we believed it to be the will of God, and as we hoped that many people would benefit from the message God wished to convey through us as His instruments of clay. Through our illnesses and difficulties God was purifying and humbling us so we could be useful instruments of His glory and the good of souls. Continued reflections from November 2009:

> My peace is gone. When I read Scripture now it accuses me rather than consoles me. The pain is 10,000 times worse than dying. It is all about love, about God's love, about loving God and others. I accept this darkness which I pray is a purgation because it is God's will. I see everything and everyone differently. I seem to be detached from everything,

except my desire to be saved, to be loved by God and to love Him, and to love and serve others. This is all God's work. I could not have achieved a tiny portion of this purification by my own efforts. This is all being done by God's light, which is blinding darkness and pain for me.

I pray with my whole heart and soul for sinners, especially those most in need of God's mercy. I want none to go to Hell even for one minute let alone eternity. I forgive everyone though it seems there is nothing to forgive. I beg for Jesus's mercy, and I will and desire to be merciful to others. Help me, Jesus and Mary, please, I am counting on you.

Jesus, I trust in You, in Your infinite mercy, which is Your greatest attribute. St. Faustina, pray for me! I prayed in the past to have St. Faustina's spiritual life, even at any cost, though I had no idea how painful this could be. I stand by my original prayer as difficult as it is, only by God's grace. I desire peace, though I surrender to the purification our Heavenly Father requires of me. Please, Jesus, help me to live my remaining time well, and in Your grace.

Interestingly I started a thirty-three day consecration to the Blessed Virgin Mary on November 5, 2009. The early part is all about gaining self-knowledge in the light of the Holy Spirit, etc. This is what I am experiencing. This is also the liturgical end of the Church year where the readings call us to prepare for our judgment, which each of us will face.

It is good to remember that night leads to day, Good Friday to Easter, death to resurrection, pain and suffering to transfigured, new, and improved bodies for all eternity.

I told Jesus that I have been humbled, that I can't carry this cross (illness) by myself. I asked Him to carry all or most for me. I asked Him to please give me peace.

I believe I was going through a *dark night* as coined by St. John of the Cross for an extended period of time. It was terrible. But I will to have Faith, Hope, Love, and so I do. These are found in the will, not the emotions. It is a decision. The truth is that, as dark as it gets, Jesus is always close to us, even closer in the darkness. This darkness is the most painful experience one can endure. One feels totally abandoned by God. One's sins and imperfections are exposed. One enters closer into God's light, which is too bright and painful for the soul. It is like coming from a dark room into a light one thousand times brighter than the sunniest day. The light actually overwhelms the eyes, causing pain and placing them in darkness. But what is really happening here is that God is giving the soul a special gift of purification, sanctifying the soul, drawing it more intimately closer to Him, pruning it so that it will be fruitful. It is the law of the cross.

Only through the gift of the cross can we advance spiritually to a significant degree. This conforms us to our savior, Jesus, who experienced the cross and abandonment before us and with us. "From noon onward, darkness came over the whole land until three in the afternoon. And about three o'clock Jesus cried out in a loud voice, 'Eli, Eli, lema sabachthani?' which means, 'My God, my God, why have you forsaken me?'" (Matthew 27:45–46). This is all God's work in the soul. Was Jesus abandoned by the Father even for a moment? No, never! But, He experienced abandonment in His human nature in the agony of darkness on the cross.

In this darkness the soul must continue to make acts of the will proclaiming his faith in the absolute truth that God loves him infinitely, and this is incontestably true. He must hand himself over unconditionally and with great confidence and trust to the certain love and mercy of God. God never changes. He always loves us. He is always ready to forgive if we seek pardon. Jesus died to save sinners, not the righteous. "I did not come to call the righteous but sinners" (Mark 2:17). The more a sinner I am, I can safely say, the more I have a claim to His mercy. "I tell you, there will be more rejoicing in heaven over one repentant sinner than over ninety-nine virtuous men who have no need of repentance" (Luke 15:7, JB). It was shortly after His cry of abandonment that Jesus expressed His complete trust in the Father, just before He died. "Jesus cried out in a loud voice, 'Father, into your hands I commend my spirit'; and when he had said this he breathed his last" (Luke 23:46).

By the way, when we are suffering from a cross it is helpful to remember that Jesus chose to go first. None of us can suffer as much as Jesus did out of love for us.

It is good in an overwhelming situation to pray often: Jesus, I trust in You. Holy Spirit, fill me and give me peace. Heavenly Father, I love You; continue to protect me, Your beloved child.

Dark nights are common in Scripture. They prepare, purify, and humble the subject to prepare him or her to be effective instruments in his or her missions given by God. Here are just a few examples.

> Now as the sun was setting Abram fell into a deep sleep, and terror seized him. Then Yahweh said to Abram, "Know this for certain, that your descendants will be exiles in a land not their own, where they will be slaves and oppressed for four hundred years. But I will pass judgement also on the nation that enslaves them and after that they will leave, with many possessions. For your part, you shall go to your fathers in peace; you shall be buried at a ripe old age. In the fourth generation they will come back here, for the wickedness of the Amorites is not yet ended." When the sun had set and darkness had fallen, there appeared a smoking furnace and a firebrand that went between the halves. That day Yahweh made a Covenant with Abram in

these terms: "To your descendants I give this land, from the wadi of Egypt to the Great River…"

Genesis 15:12–19 (JB)

Here, Abram, who is later to be renamed Abraham by God, went through his dark night. It is described in this scripture passage by referring to terror seizing Abram, and darkness approaching with the sun setting. He is given some bad news about his descendants being exiles, slaves, and oppressed for four hundred years; however, God adds that He will free them, and that Abram will live to a ripe old age. After Abram had passed through this darkness he was purified and prepared to receive and make a covenant with God. God had very big plans for Abram, but he needed to be purified first through the cross, like you and me.

There is the psalmist who writes, "Wretched, slowly dying since my youth, I bore your terrors-now I am exhausted; anger overwhelmed me, you destroyed me with your terrors which, like a flood, were round me, all day long, all together closing in on me. You have turned my friends and neighbours against me, now darkness is my one companion left" (Psalm 88:15–18, JB). It is intriguing to see how often the word darkness, or some derivative, is used in Scripture to describe *the sense* of the absence of God. Keep in mind that this is only a sense, because God is actually at all times present with His love. The subject in this psalm suffers greatly in soul and spirit. The truth is that God never abandons any of us even for one moment of our lives. But He does mysteriously permit us to experience a sense of the loss of God, as a means of purification to draw us closer to Him.

Then there is the greatest apostle of all time, St. Paul. He originally went by the name Saul. At the very moment of his conversion he went through something of a dark night to prepare him for his awesome mission of bringing Jesus to the Gentiles. This was only the first of numerous, painful crosses for St. Paul.

Acts 9:1–22 (JB):

> Meanwhile Saul was still breathing threats to slaughter the
> Lord's disciples. He had gone to the high priest and asked
> for letters addressed to the synagogues in Damascus that
> would authorise him to arrest and take to Jerusalem any
> followers of the Way, men or women, that he could find.
> Suddenly, while he was traveling to Damascus and just
> before he reached the city, there came a light from heaven
> all round him. He fell to the ground, and then he heard
> a voice saying, "Saul, Saul, why are you persecuting me?"
> "Who are you, Lord?" he asked, and the voice answered, "I
> am Jesus, and you are persecuting me."

This, by the way, is a beautiful insight into the Mystical Body of
Jesus Christ wherein Jesus takes on our sufferings and divinizes
them. We see that Saul was persecuting members of the Church,
in that Jesus identifies with them as being the one persecuted,
even though He is standing at the right hand of the Father.[6]

"'Get up now and go to the city, and you will be told what you
have to do.' The men traveling with Saul stood there speechless,
for though they heard the voice, they could see no one. Saul got
up from the ground, but even with his eyes wide open he could
see nothing at all, and they had to lead him into Damascus by
hand." We see that when we are exposed to the light of Christ, the
extreme brightness becomes darkness to us, at least for a period of
time. So never fear. The darkness will become light again for those
God has especially chosen to experience the darkness of his light
in a bountiful way. This darkness is transforming. It will be seen as
nothing but a blessing throughout eternity when we realize what
we have gained by this cross.

We also see here how Saul surrendered to be led by the hand,
to go blindly into the city, without even knowing the purpose. This
must have been difficult for him. We are often called to take one

step at a time in God's providential plan for us, not knowing what the next step will bring. This way we learn to live in the present and to trust more in Jesus.

"For three days he was without his sight and took neither food nor drink." So he eventually came back into the light and was able to see. It is interesting that there is a type of death and resurrection, Good Friday and Easter, as Jesus died and was in the tomb for three days before he rose. We also see how Saul fasted, which was his own effort to be purified. I am certain that the most efficacious part of his cross was the part that God sent him.

> A disciple called Ananias who lived in Damascus had a vision in which he heard the Lord say to him, "Ananias!" When he replied, "Here I am Lord", the Lord said, "You must go to Straight Street and ask at the house of Judas for someone called Saul who comes from Tarsus. At this moment he is praying, having had a vision of a man called Ananias coming in and laying hands on him to give him back his sight." When he heard that, Ananias said, "Lord, several people have told me about this man and all the harm he has been doing to your saints in Jerusalem. He only comes here because he holds a warrant from the chief priests to arrest everybody who invokes your name." The Lord replied, "You must go all the same, because this man is my chosen instrument to bring my name before pagans and pagan kings and before the people of Israel; I myself will show him how much he himself must suffer for my name."

We see how Saul was chosen, as we ourselves are *chosen* for a particular mission. This is based on no merit of our own. We note that Saul was a major persecutor of the Church. The Lord Jesus saw not what he had been, but what he would become...a *masterpiece*. He looks at us in the same way at every moment with

His loving countenance. Not only does God forgive the worse sinners, even enemies of His Church, but He makes them His *chosen instruments*, like the great St Paul.

We who suffer have been chosen. Let us always unite our sufferings to Christ as we suffer for His name to bring glory to God and assistance to our neighbors. May we do what we can to serve God and others. Lord, help me to live this personally!

"Then Ananias went and he entered the house, and at once laid his hands on Saul and said, 'Brother Saul, I have been sent by the Lord who appeared to you on your way here so that you may recover your sight and be filled with the Holy Spirit.'" Like Ananias, each of us is sent by Jesus to fulfill our particular mission. God himself relied on Ananias so that Paul might be healed and filled with the Holy Spirit. He relies on us to bring the Holy Spirit to others.

"Immediately it was as though scales fell from Saul's eyes and he could see again. So he was baptized there and then, and after taking some food he regained his strength." Paul was lifted out of the darkness and into the light by the Holy Spirit. When this happens to us we begin to become givers; we become pourers. We gain strength through the Holy Spirit. That grace is not to be stagnant. Saul regained his strength and used it to become a great, sacrificial apostle. Contrary to what we might think on a strictly human level, the more we give of ourselves, the more strength we receive.

"After he has spent only a few days with the disciples in Damascus, he began preaching in the synagogues, 'Jesus is the son of God.'" We see how Saul wasted no time to engage in his mission.

> All his hearers were amazed. "Surely," they said, "This is the man who organized the attack in Jerusalem against the people who invoke this name, and who came here for the sole purpose of arresting them to have them tried by the chief priests?" Saul's power increased steadily, and he was

able to throw the Jewish colony at Damascus into complete confusion by the way he demonstrated that Jesus was the Christ.

When we repent, accept Jesus's mercy, embrace Him, and become apostles with the talents and mission He gave us, we receive power. This is not a merely human power. It is a supernatural power that comes from the Holy Spirit. This is not a power we take pride in, but a power that drives and invigorates us. We are no longer focused on ourselves, but on others. We become joyful deep down. We often gain energy and a sense of health that we did not have before, because the more we give the more we receive. May each of us do all that is necessary to receive this power for the glory of God and the salvation of His children, for whom He has given us a responsibility.

Another apropos example of one experiencing darkness and eventually being delivered into the light is contained in the third chapter of Lamentations.

> I am the man familiar with misery under the rod of his anger; I am the one he has driven and forced to walk in darkness, and without any light. Against me alone he turns his hand, again and again, all day long. He has wasted my flesh and skin away, has broken my bones. He has make a yoke for me, has encircled my head with weariness. He has forced me to dwell in darkness with the dead of long ago...
>
> Lamentation 3:1–6 (JB)

The lamentation continues, but eventually turns to hope.

> And now I say, "My strength is gone, that hope which came from Yahweh." Brooding on my anguish and affliction is gall and wormwood. My spirit ponders it continually and

sinks within me. That is what I shall tell my heart and so recover hope: the favours of Yahweh are not all past, his kindnesses are not exhausted; every morning they are renewed; great is his faithfulness. "My portion is Yahweh" says my soul "and so I will hope in him." Yahweh is good to those who trust him, to the soul that searches for him. It is good to wait in silence for Yahweh to save.

Lamentations 3:18–26 (JB)

Yes, we can count on God to always arrange everything for our ultimate good. If we search for the Lord, He will be found. When we wait in silence for Him to save, we grow in our trust in Him.

And we also have King David speaking of his dark night and eventual deliverance:

I waited, waited for the LORD;/ who bent down and heard my cry,/ Drew me out of the pit of destruction,/ out of the mud of the swamp,/ Set my feet upon rock,/ steadied my steps,/ And put a new song in my mouth,/ a hymn to our God./ Many shall look on in awe/ and they shall trust in the LORD.

Psalm 40:2–4

Jesus, please never permit me, like Judas, to exercise the gift of my free will disastrously by betraying You and by not seeking Your mercy when I do fall, especially after all the tremendous graces that You have showered upon me through no merit of my own. "So he took the morsel and left at once. And it was night" (John 13:30). I have great confidence that You will protect me from entering the true *night*, the true darkness, which is separation from You.

Perhaps the greatest adversities, which our infinitely wise Father uses to bring a tremendous good out of, in order to purify us and to help others in His mysterious ways, are darkness, abandonment, and staring death in the face. Joseph of the Old Testament is a perfect example of this. He is truly a Christ figure; and we are all called to be other Christ's. Many are familiar with his amazing story. Joseph was a shepherd of the flock (like Jesus, the Good Shepherd). He was also a dreamer. May we all be dreamers! May we never give up on our God-inspired dreams, and on His beautiful dream for us.

Joseph's brothers were jealous of him. They turned on him, and threw him into a well to die. Then they decided to sell him into slavery for twenty silver pieces (see Genesis 37). They abandoned him, the very ones who should have been his most loyal supporters, such as happened to Jesus, the truly innocent one. "And they all deserted him and ran away" (Mark 14:50–51, JB). The price of a slave had gone up by the time of Jesus:

> Then one of the Twelve, who was called Judas Iscariot, went to the chief priests and said, "What are you willing to give me if I hand him over to you?" They paid him thirty pieces of silver, and from that time on he looked for an opportunity to hand him over.
>
> Matthew 26:14–16

In Egypt Joseph was falsely accused by his master's wife and thrown in the darkness of jail and imprisonment. He was beyond doubt in a dire, disastrous situation, with outwardly little hope to hold on to. But God always has His good plan. We always have hope.

Joseph later interpreted Pharaoh's dream. His wisdom and prophecy were recognized, and he was appointed governor of the whole land (see Genesis 39–41). Joseph prudently stored food throughout Egypt in anticipation of a severe famine, which he had prophesied. Eventually, when there was famine throughout the whole world, Joseph came to the rescue. Joseph's entire family was saved through the sharing of the food he had stocked away. Joseph revealed himself to his brothers and treated them with mercy, those very ones who had sold him into slavery, and Joseph made this statement:

> God sent me before you to make sure that your race would have survivors in the land and to save your lives, many lives at that. So it was not you who sent me here but God, and he has made me father to Pharaoh, lord of all his household and administrator of the whole land of Egypt.

> Genesis 45:7–8 (JB)

Joseph later added: "The evil you planned to do me has by God's design been turned to good, that he might bring about, as indeed he has, the deliverance of a numerous people" (Genesis 50:20–21, JB). God's design? How can he say that? Wasn't it his brothers' sin that caused him so much pain? Well, yes, his brothers did evil. God never wants evil, but when it happens only He can, and always does, bring a tremendous good out of it—and that includes our cancer and other adversities. May we never doubt this! Our loving Father is seeing to everything for our good, no exceptions! Look at all the fruits of Joseph's crosses, how holy he became, and the numerous people who were delivered from famine. Moreover our crosses are sanctifying us, and are helping Jesus to deliver/redeem numerous souls. What a privilege!

So with great confidence we continue forward in God's grace in our lives, our mission…"relying on the power of God who has saved us and called us to be holy—not because of anything we ourselves have done but for his own purpose and by his own grace" (2 Timothy 1:8–9, JB).

Once again we find comforting assurance in the following dynamic Scripture promise: "We know that by turning everything to their good God co-operates with all those who love him, with all those that he has called according to his purpose" (Romans 8:28, JB). We cannot see in advance everything good that will come of our adversities, many of which can seem to us to be unfair, or to serve no good purpose, and which are very painful. Like St. Paul in his great mission, we are called to take one step in darkness at a time in total abandonment, trusting Jesus, who is holding us by the hand through the darkness at every step. "Saul got up from the ground, but even with his eyes wide open he could see nothing at all, and they had to lead him into Damascus by the hand" (Acts 9: 8–9, JB). Jesus, I trust in You!

HEALING
FOR SOUL AND SPIRIT

"May the God of peace himself make you perfectly holy and may you entirely, spirit, soul, and body, be preserved blameless for the coming of our Lord Jesus Christ. The one who calls you is faithful, and he will also accomplish it" (1 Thessalonians 5:23–24).

October 2010: I have been receiving Campath along with Rituxan immunotherapy for my leukemia. My body has reacted quite badly in response to the Campath. I ran fevers for approximately five weeks fluctuating between no fever to low grade to 101 degrees plus, though the fevers gradually became reduced and of lesser duration after the first few weeks. I lost almost 20 pounds during this time. At one point I felt I could not endure one more day of these fevers.

Edited excerpts from my diary, October 13, 2010:

I've been through two weeks of agony and darkness. I have been running fevers, experiencing chills, drenching sweats, headaches, hallucinations, feeling as if I was living in a fog or a tunnel, coughing, having no appetite, smells of food making me sick, feeling terrible, and literally feeling like I was dying. I looked terrible. It was hard to see how I could go on like this much longer. On October 12, 2010, I prayed to the Blessed Virgin Mary that if it was in accord with God's most holy and perfect will, my fever would end today, as I did not feel I had the strength for another day. That morning I received the Anointing of the Sick by Father Ildephonse. I went to Northwestern for the Campath as usual, and this time they gave me my first round of Rituxan with a dose of steroids. My hematologist/oncologist thought that steroids might help the fever. Sure enough, all things combined—the Blessed Mother's intercession, the grace of God, and the help of the medical community—my fever was gone and has remained gone since then.

It is amazing how much recovered I feel in one day. My platelets are up to 88,000. Praise the Lord. It was as if being reborn again, but more spiritually. I came out of the tunnel. Last night, I went into the bathroom after severe night sweats, and I said to the devil, "You cannot have me; you cannot stop me—God is my Father!" At this moment, my entire organism trembled violently, my hands were raised, I sobbed, and I prayed so deeply. It was as if God was making me aware of how He is filling me with His love and His grace, but I do not have the capacity for it. It was so overwhelming, but so powerful and beautiful. I could see how God is so wonderful, and that He is my All. I can see all people and things clearly for what they are, so beautiful, but without being attached in any way. I believe that when I am praying for others there is great efficacy there, by the grace of God. What beautiful gifts from God have arisen from my sufferings! "Yours has been a kind of suffering that God approves....To suffer in God's way means changing for the better and leaves no regrets, but to suffer as the world knows suffering brings death. Just look at what suffering in God's way has brought you:

what keenness, what explanations, what indignation, what alarm!" (2 Corinthians 7:9–11, JB).

I had these experiences, which I believe were gifts from God, numerous times through the night and day when I would just think of God or some manifestation of Him. There is a deep sense of God's presence and love, and a deep trembling of body and spirit. When I pray for others at these moments, the prayers seem very powerful. I also had this experience right after Communion (receiving Jesus in the consecrated Host). I cannot make the experience start, but I can move myself out of the experience when I need to move on to a responsibility.

I pray that I will not lose the graces and the insights, love, and detachments that I have been gifted with through no merit on my part. These gifts have been acquired through so much pain.

"Think of what Christ suffered in this life, and then arm yourselves with the same resolution that he had: anyone who in this life has bodily suffering has broken with sin, because for the rest of his life on earth he is not ruled by human passions but only by the will of God" (1 Peter 4:1–3, JB).

God has thrown some consolations my way as He knows what a weakling I am. I gratefully accept them as only He knows what is best for my soul at any given moment. I am certain that this particular gift of consolations is not going to last. God is not to be found in these emotional experiences. They are the things of God, not God Himself. But God gives these gifts as He sees fit at the perfect times according to His most perfect providence so as to bolster us for whatever comes next, so that we will remain *faithful and true* as Jesus was and is. "Its rider was [called] 'Faithful and True'" (Revelation 19:11).

These consolations are a gift from God to strengthen us, and to move us to love more. "The feelings only serve as stimulants to love."[7] Most importantly, we need to keep our equilibrium through times of both darkness and comfort, knowing God loves us and supports us at all times—though in a sense we might say that He is closer to us in times of darkness because it is so costly to us to keep our faith and trust at those times.

And if we seldom or never experience consolations from God, despite our love for Him, and our prayers and the offering of our suffering to Him, if we experience only darkness and dryness, take heart, because we have been specially chosen to live the example of Jesus on the cross more intimately. The longsuffering soul who feels abandoned, who experiences this seeming constant darkness, has indeed been chosen by our Father in heaven for this higher, more efficacious suffering that helps many souls find their salvation and gives great glory to God. "My God, my God, why have you forsaken me?" (Matthew 27:46).

God is always bringing such tremendously great good out of everything. Thank You, Abba. Thank You, Holy Spirit. Thank You, Jesus. Thank you, Mary, for your powerful and wonderful intercession.

Edited excerpts from my diary:

> October 24, 2010: I have been broken in body, mind, soul, and spirit, brought low to the bottom by our merciful Father. I know this is a special grace because by this unbelievably painful and purging experience, God had brought me low enough that He can now lift me up to Himself. I am presently often overcome with God's presence and love, which so overwhelms me physically, emotionally, mentally, and in the spirit that I tremble uncontrollably and pray wordless prayers in union with our Heavenly Father. This is in spite of my many faults that I receive this tremendous grace. I believe that I have been given the gift of a great power of intercession for others in my prayer especially at these moments which seem to come frequently, for

example, whenever I think of God or His manifestations in some way.

October 31, 2010: A couple days ago I came to Psalm 60 in the *Liturgy of the Hours*.[8] In my *Jerusalem Bible* it states, "God, you have rejected us, broken us" (Psalm 60: 1, JB). I have used the term *broken*, that God had *broken* me, numerous times in recent weeks in my prayer and in conversations with my wife, Kathleen. I did not know this was scriptural at the time. I was not saying "broken" in a negative sense, but rather proclaiming a reality from the depths of my soul and spirit. Everything that God permits is enfolded in His most perfect providence, and is a gift. The experience of being broken by God is painful, but it is among the most wonderful gifts I have ever received as there is no other way He could have gifted me with such union with Him as I have experienced. I praise the Lord for bringing me so low and breaking me that He might lift me up, purify, renew, and sanctify me so that I can be more effective in my life for His glory and for souls, and so I can grow in humility (I have a long way to go!). God can only accomplish efficacious, momentous, lasting things through humble souls.

My illness has brought so many tremendous, deep blessings that cannot be acquired any other way. The cross is truly a gift, as difficult as it is for us to understand and endure on a human level. "The message of the cross is foolishness to those who are perishing, but to us who are being saved it is the power of God" (1 Corinthians 1:18). The cross is God's power at work transforming us into the people we are meant to be. We are being healed in many ways by the cross.

Be assured that your cross is blooming with the fruit of blessings. If you cannot see these blessings in your own life, ask the Holy Spirit to give you the supernatural sight to recognize these gifts. They are there. God loves you so much that there is no other possibility. *This is certain.*

The gift of the cross heals us, purifies us, and amends for sin. It prepares us to repent and accept the gift of redemption. Shortly after I was diagnosed I went to a General Confession where I did my best to confess all the sins of my lifetime. Now this would probably take the average reader about ten to twenty minutes. It took me three-and-a-half hours as I have broken every commandment in virtually every way possible in the course of my life. My confession may have qualified the priest, who had the patience of a saint, for canonization. Now if all my sins, and they are many, can be forgiven and forgotten by God, then yours most certainly will be forgiven and forgotten if you seek the infinite mercy of Jesus. "I have brushed away your offenses like a cloud,/ your sins like a mist;/ return to me, for I have redeemed you" (Isaiah 44:22).

Can our all-knowing God actually forget our sins? Yes, only because He chooses to do so, and promises that He will. When we repent, our sins are blotted out, erased. "I it is, I it is, who must blot out everything and not remember your sins" (Isaiah 43:25, JB).

The following quote is from the Diary of St. Faustina Kowalska. These are the words of Jesus to her to be shared with us:

> (Let) the greatest sinners place their trust in My mercy. They have the right before others to trust in the abyss of My mercy. My daughter, write about My mercy towards tormented souls. Souls that make an appeal to My mercy delight me. To such souls I grant even more graces than they ask. I cannot punish even the greatest sinner if he makes an appeal to My compassion, but on the contrary, I justify him in My unfathomable and inscrutable mercy. Write: before I come as a just Judge, I first open the wide

door of My mercy. He who refuses to pass through the door of My mercy must pass through the door of My justice.

Diary 1146[9]

What solace we can take from these words! Those of us, like me, who are the greatest sinners, have the right before others to trust in the abyss of Christ's mercy!

God our infinitely merciful Father is always seeking us out, ready to forgive, ready to pour His infinite mercy upon us. This reality is portrayed beautifully in the well-known "Prodigal Son" passage in Luke 15:11–24: "Then he said, 'A man had two sons, and the younger son said to his father, "Father, give me the share of your estate that should come to me." So the father divided the property between them.'" Let's look at this from the perspective that we are the younger son. The younger son takes his share of the inheritance which, in fact, is not yet his. This is what we do when we try to make our life on earth into heaven. This is an impossible aspiration and will only leave us empty and unhappy, because only God can satisfy us.

We make a god (who is fake, deceiving, little, and powerless) out of many things including power, sex, material possessions, pleasure, ego. We end up miserable. We end up stuffed, sated, and sick as a result of our self-centered overconsumption in life. "After a few days, the younger son collected all his belongings." The younger son collected all his belongings in the way that we tend to cling to our materialism, "and set off to a distant country where he squandered his inheritance on a life of dissipation." Note that the younger son left the father behind. We tend to leave God our Father behind, seeking our happiness in things that will never satisfy. We tend to squander our inheritance, which is our loving God Himself. We end up lost and lonely when we are away from our Loving Father in what feels like a distant country. It is also like a distant country because it seems that no one speaks our language; no one can truly understand us. We have left the peace of home behind.

Only our Heavenly Father can fill our ache to be fully happy. We tend to place our securities in things, things that cannot save, things that disappoint, things that do not fill our emptiness, things that cannot take us and that we cannot take with us into eternity. We are truly secure in only one place, in God's hands, and that is where we always are unless we choose to pull away. Even then He seeks us. "Take this as certain."[10]

"When he had freely spent everything, a severe famine struck that country and he found himself in dire need." Yes, we tend to spend ourselves on inferior things, and we end up utterly spent. We end up suffering famine, we are starved for love, because we have chosen to separate ourselves from our Father who loves us with an *overshadowing love* (see Mark 9:7). We find that the things we placed our security in only left us all the more in dire need. Only God has the capacity to accommodate our security placed in Him. He will never let us down. He is *faithful and true.*

> Then I saw the heavens opened, and there was a white horse; its rider was [called] "Faithful and True." He judges and wages war in righteousness. His eyes were [like] a fiery flame, and on his head were many diadems. He had a name inscribed that no one knows except himself. He wore a cloak that had been dipped in blood, and his name was called the Word of God.
>
> Revelation 19:11–13

Yes, Jesus, the Word of God, loves us so much that He became man so He could shed His blood for us unto death. And oh, His look! His penetrating look of Love with eyes on fire with Love for us, for me, for you! He chooses to wear a cloak dipped in His own

Blood as a reminder to us and to His Father of His faithfulness in loving us. Is there any faithfulness to compare with this?

Returning to the Prodigal Son from Luke 15:11–24: "So he hired himself out to one of the local citizens who sent him to his farm to tend the swine. And he longed to eat his fill of the pods in which the swine fed." Yes, when we separate ourselves from God we find ourselves starving, drained, and empty. We find our dignity reduced to that of swine, longing to glut ourselves with whatever inferior things we have become attached to. Our dignity has been cheapened. We turn to others to try to fill this void, but they alone cannot save. They alone do not have the capacity to love us as our Father of Mercies in heaven. "But nobody gave him any." Nobody has the capacity to furnish us what we truly need to be filled.

"Coming to his senses he thought, 'How many of my father's hired workers have more than enough food to eat, but here am I, dying from hunger.'" Because He is such a wise and merciful Father, He permits us, sometimes the hard way, to learn how empty and lost we are without Him. We find ourselves literally dying from hunger for God. We are now prepared to notice and be drawn to others who have remained with or have come to the Father. We see the light of Christ shining through them. We admire their peace. They have more than enough to fill them, because they have God.

"I shall get up and go to my father and I shall say to him, 'Father, I have sinned against heaven and against you. I no longer deserve to be called your son; treat me as you would treat one of your hired workers.'" What a beautiful, truthful, and humble profession of contrition. It seems that most of us tend to have to descend very low into the darkness before we can come to the realization of how much our Father loves us, how we can only be happy with Him. We do need to exercise our free will to seek His mercy, but it is always available.

God our Father is actually continually seeking us out, but He will never retract His gift of free will. Without free will we would be incapable of loving, as love involves a free choice, a willingness to sacrifice for the other. God will never tamper with this fundamental gift, even though He must risk the terrible and real possibility that we will use it to make wrong and harmful choices, even at the horrifying risk that we will abuse our freedom unto the eternal loss of our soul. This is one of the answers to why God permits so much evil in the world. He does not force. He wants our authentic love, as weak as it may be.

The supreme marvel of God's sublime strategy is profoundly expressed by St. Augustine with these words: "He judged it better to draw good out of evil than not to permit evil to exist."[11] God does not want draftees against their will. He wants zealous, loving, committed volunteers fighting for souls in His Kingdom. He will never institute the draft in His Kingdom, though He is known to use extraordinary means to move the hearts of souls, like He did with St. Paul, literally knocking him off his horse to help him. We must choose to accept His healing embrace. We must resolve to seek Him out, even when confused and mistakenly feeling that we might be rejected. Our Father of Mercies will never reject us!

[The prodigal son then] "got up and went back to his father. While he was still a long way off, his father caught sight of him, and was filled with compassion. He ran to his son, embraced him and kissed him." See, the father had spent his days longingly looking out on the horizon, hoping for a glimpse of his son returning. Our Father in heaven is constantly looking for us and sees us when we are still a long way off. Note that it was the father who acted first, the father who was filled with compassion and ran to his son. It was the father who embraced his son and kissed him before the son said a word. This mercy and forgiveness is always awaiting us as sons and daughters of our Merciful Father. No matter what! Yes, I said no matter what!

"His son said to him, 'Father, I have sinned against heaven and against you; I no longer deserve to be called your son.'" How does the father express his love and exhibit the forgiveness and mercy he has already given to his son? "But his father ordered his servants, 'Quickly bring the finest robe and put it on him; put a ring on his finger and sandals on his feet. Take the fattened calf and slaughter it. Then let us celebrate with a feast.'" I think we often think that God our Father will treat us in the human way we might treat others. We think: Yes, He might forgive, but grudgingly and perhaps, like us, getting into "I told you so." No! We see that the father treats his son like royalty, without any reference to the sins that have been forgiven and forgotten and will never be mentioned again.

There is a celebration, and they celebrate with a feast. Clothing the son with a robe represents the white garment we are clothed with in Baptism, wherein we become incorporated into Christ as priest, prophet, and king. "The *anointing with sacred chrism*, perfumed oil consecrated by the bishop, signifies the gift of the Holy Spirit to the newly baptized, who has become a Christian, that is, one 'anointed' by the Holy Spirit, incorporated into Christ who is anointed priest, prophet, and king"[12] (CCC 1241). We are transformed into the common priesthood of all the faithful (including bishops and priests who are ordained into the profound and oh so indispensible ministerial priesthood; as well as deacons who "are ministers ordained for tasks of service of the Church" CCC 1596[13]) metaphorically wearing priestly rings, prophets wearing sandals to help us travel to bring the good news to souls, robes demonstrating our royalty as kings.

> Christ, high priest and unique mediator, has made of the Church "a kingdom, priests for his God and Father."
> [14] The whole community of believers is, as such, priestly. The faithful exercise their baptismal priesthood through their participation, each according to his own vocation, in

Christ's mission as priest, prophet, and king. Through the sacraments of Baptism and Confirmation the faithful are "consecrated to be...a holy priesthood."[15]

CCC 1546

There is something else happening here as well. There is no remission of sin without the shedding of blood (see Hebrews 9:22). We see that the fattened calf is slaughtered, its blood is shed. The father's servants participate in this feast by consuming the calf. This points to the Eucharist, where we in the Catholic Church consume the flesh of the innocent Lamb of God, Jesus. It is through the amazing love of the Father in giving His only Son over to His passion and death for the forgiveness of our sins that we are saved, that we can be forgiven. And those of us who were dead in sin come to life again, as did Jesus Who went to death in order to put death to death and came to life in His resurrection. "Because this son of mine was dead and has come to life again; he was lost and has been found." We are found and healed by God our Father. What could be more beautiful? All of heaven and earth rejoice when a sinner repents and receives the always ready and available mercy of God. "Then the celebration began." All are called to seek and receive as a gift God's readily available mercy and forgiveness. Our Heavenly Father is waiting expectantly for us as in the parable of the Prodigal Son.

As a matter of fact, if one had committed every possible sin ever committed from the beginning of time to the end of the world, including the vilest imaginable, these sins would still be finite, amounting to infinitely less than one drop in all the oceans of the world compared with the infinite sacrifice and mercy of Jesus. Jesus is God and therefore infinite; His sacrifice was consequently infinite and able to consume and obliterate all the sins of the world as if they were only a single grain of sand in all the beaches of the world. He came not to save only those who live good lives with

90

only a few minor sins (as if such a person exists), but especially those big sinners like me. The greatest attribute of Jesus is mercy. St. Faustina quotes Jesus's private revelation to her in her Diary, "Proclaim that mercy is the greatest attribute of God. All the works of My hands are crowned with mercy." (Diary 301)[16]

Never despair of it supposedly being too late for repentance and to receive God's mercy. God does not act according to our narrow ways. It is never too late, even if we have been idle about the things of God all of our lives! We can always get a fresh start in the present moment. Praised be God for His marvelous generosity!

HEALING IN BODY

"I must fulfill the vows I made you, God; I shall pay you my thank-offerings, for you have rescued me from Death to walk in the presence of God in the light of the living" (Psalm 56:12–13, JB).

Edited excerpts from my diary:

> May 25, 2010: Today I received more dire news from my hematologist/oncologist regarding my life expectancy without a stem-cell transplant or perhaps the clinical trial I am interested in. She also called me later in the day to tell me my platelets dropped further to 29,000. Jesus, I trust in You! Mary, please arrange everything for me. Jesus, please, have mercy on me and all sinners, and on all the souls in purgatory. I opened at random to Jeremiah 30:17 (JB): "But I will restore you to health and heal your wounds—it is Yahweh who speaks."
>
> On October 28, 2010, in the evening I went to the emergency room. To make a long story short, Kathleen and I were up all night in the emergency room. I was diagnosed with a pulmonary embolism (blood clot) in the lower lobe of the right lung, and pneumonia in the left lung. I was admitted and kept overnight on October 29, but sent home on October 30, Saturday. My pulse had been running fast

at about 120 beats per minute for weeks, but it came down to about the 90s when I was discharged. Today it was at 79.

So I have these two serious conditions, but I am doing quite well by the grace of God. A pulmonary embolism can be fatal, but mine is apparently small and was caught early. I will be on blood thinners, daily self-administered Fragmin shots, for many months to come, while we hope and pray, God willing, that my platelet count stays high enough so I can keep taking it. The Fragmin does not heal the pulmonary embolism but prevents it from growing bigger, while the body goes to work on dissolving it, which generally takes about two to three months.

Psalm 60 wraps up with: "help us in this hour of crisis, the help that man can give is worthless. With God among us we shall fight like heroes, he will trample on our enemies" (Psalm 60:11–12, JB).

October 31, 2010: This morning I opened at random to Exodus 23:20–27 (JB), which reads in part: "I myself will send an angel before you to guard you as you go and to bring you to the place that I have prepared...My angel will go before you and lead you...You are to worship Yahweh your God, and I shall bless your bread and water, and remove sickness from among you. In your land no woman will miscarry, none will be barren. I shall give you your full term of life." Alleluia! Praise the Lord!

"When it was evening, they brought him many who were possessed by demons, and he drove out the spirits by a word and cured all the sick, to fulfill what had been said by Isaiah the prophet:/ "He took away our infirmities/ and bore our diseases"" (Matthew 8:16–17). Our body is a temple of the Holy Spirit. Our body is good.

Jesus can still cure the sick, and He does in many cases. It is totally within His power. All power belongs to Him. As God, He can heal us with a *nod*. We must have great confidence in Him!

"They may put their trust in their weapons and their exploits," he said; "but our confidence is in almighty God, who is able with a nod to overthrow both those marching on us and the whole world with them" (2 Maccabees 8:18–19, JB).

Shortly after I was diagnosed with leukemia, in fact ten days later, October 29, 2009, I woke up with an obscure phrase running through my mind: "My tent is folded (or pulled) up." Where did this come from? One might think that I am a Bible scholar (or perhaps not!) because I am referring so often to Scripture. I am not. I simply read and pray with Scripture daily, by the grace of God, as I have done for many years. However, I could not recognize this phrase, and was unsure whether it even was Scripture. As I often do, I opened my Bible at random for my morning prayer and came upon these very words: "My tent is pulled up, and thrown away" (Isaiah 38:12, JB). (This is the translation of my Jerusalem Bible which I usually use in prayer.) With the New American Bible quoted often in this book, the translation is: "My dwelling, like a shepherd's tent,/ is struck down and borne away from me." This did not sound very encouraging! However, I went on to read the entire passage, Isaiah 38:1–20.

This tells the story of King Hezekiah. "When Hezekiah was mortally ill, the prophet Isaiah, son of Amoz, came and said to him, 'Thus says the LORD: Put your house in order, for you are about to die; you shall not recover.'" This was still not sounding very encouraging to me!

> Then Hezekiah turned his face to the wall and prayed to the LORD....Then the word of the LORD came to Isaiah: "Go, tell Hezekiah: Thus says the LORD, the God of your father David: I have heard your prayer and seen your tears. I will heal you: in three days you shall go up to the LORD's temple; I will add fifteen years to your life."

Whew! Now I was much more encouraged.

Yes, God was able to heal Hezekiah instantaneously simply by His own power. He, however, chose to use a medical, physical means to heal him. "Isaiah then ordered a poultice of figs to be taken and applied to the boil, that he might recover." This sounds to me like the illness might have been cancer.

Hezekiah goes on to proclaim a beautiful canticle to the Lord where he begins by lamenting his illness and imminent death:

> "Once I said,/ 'In the noontime of life I must depart!/ To the gates of the nether world I shall be consigned/ for the rest of my years.'/ I said, 'I shall see the LORD no more/ in the land of the living./ No longer shall I behold my fellow men/ among those who dwell in the world.'/ My dwelling, like a shepherd's tent,/ is struck down and borne away from me;/ You have folded up my life,/ like a weaver who severs the last thread."

This beautiful canticle concludes with King Hezekiah proclaiming his healing and giving glory to God:

> Those live whom the LORD protects;/ yours...the life of my spirit./ You have given me health and life;/ thus is my bitterness transformed into peace./ You have preserved my life/ from the pit of destruction,/ When you cast behind your back/ all my sins/.... The living, the living give you thanks,/ as I do today./ Fathers declare to their sons,/ O God, your faithfulness./ The LORD is our savior;/ we shall sing to stringed instruments/ In the house of the LORD/ all the days of our life.

Now does this spiritual experience of mine mean that I will be healed physically? Only God knows, though King Hezekiah was healed physically. There are diverse ways and means God uses to heal, though He is definitely at work healing each of us, as long as we don't obstinately exercise our free will by turning our back on Him, turning our back on Love. Do I want to be healed physically? Yes, of course, I love my life; but I can also truly say with the aid of God's grace that what I want most is God's will. If His will includes a physical healing for me, may He be praised. If it does not, may He be praised. May He be praised in all ways, at all times. I am confident that when I turn to Jesus for strength, He is with me and seeing to the best for me at all times whether this includes a physical healing or not. Only He knows what is best.

And Jesus makes everything easy for us when we turn to Him. "Come to me, all you who labor and are burdened, and I will give you rest. Take my yoke upon you and learn from me, for I am meek and humble of heart; and you will find rest for yourselves. For my yoke is easy, and my burden light" (Matthew 11:28–30). Jesus, I trust in You!

I believe that when God gives a special spiritual gift or insight it is sometimes not meant to be kept to ourselves but to be shared with others for their good. In fact, the insight may be intended more for the benefit of another, or many others, more so than the initial recipient. Therefore it is my prayer that the reader will be much encouraged by the story of King Hezekiah. His story of hope is worth coming back to often for encouragement.

When Jesus walked the earth in His public ministry we know that He was constantly healing the sick.

> He went around all of Galilee, teaching in their synagogues, proclaiming the gospel of the kingdom, and curing every disease and illness among the people. His fame spread to all of Syria, and they brought to him all who were sick with various diseases and racked with pain, those who were possessed, lunatics, and paralytics, and he cured them.
>
> Matthew 4:23–24

Jesus loves us. He created our bodies, which are good. But what He is most concerned with in the long run is our eternal salvation. Even those He healed eventually died. I myself have been healed many times by Jesus when I could have died. But one thing is certain—I will one day die as will you. We will in fact be reunited with our glorious bodies at the final judgment for all eternity. In heaven there will be no more pain or sickness. "No one who dwells there will say, 'I am sick';/ the people who live there will be forgiven their guilt" (Isaiah 33:24).

It is also good to keep in mind that our physical realities are truly signs, as well as spiritual realities. Illnesses and diseases, as real as they are, also represent sin. Sin racks us with pain in our soul and spirit.

There truly exist fallen angels, demons who hate us beyond our comprehension, and who are working to destroy us. There are true cases of demonic possession today, and more often demonic oppression. When we get caught up in sin without repenting and turning to Jesus for His mercy and protection, we are placing ourselves at risk from the demonic.

I believe the paralytic healed by Jesus in both body and soul, as referred to in Mark 2:1–12, also and most significantly applies to the spiritual realm where we can become paralyzed, powerless, and unable to accomplish any lasting good when we are enslaved to sin. Fortunately this is easily remedied by turning to Jesus in repentance and receiving His always readily available grace and mercy. "When Jesus saw their faith, he said to the paralytic, 'Child, your sins are forgiven'" (Mark 2:5). This gospel passage also refers to the power of intercessory prayer and action. Jesus refers to *their* faith, not the faith of the paralytic. Why they? He is referring to the faith of the four men who interceded for the paralyzed man. They stopped at nothing, even opening up a hole in the roof to bring him to Jesus to be healed in both body and, more importantly, in soul. "Many gathered together so that there was no longer room for them, not even around the door, and he preached the word to them. They came bringing to him a paralytic carried by four men. Unable to get near Jesus because of the crowd, they opened up the roof above him. After they had broken through, they let down the mat on which the paralytic was lying."

And, yes, the paralytic was also healed in body.

> "Which is easier, to say to the paralytic, 'Your sins are forgiven,' or to say, 'Rise, pick up your mat and walk?' But that you may know that the Son of Man has authority to forgive sins on earth—he said to the paralytic, "I say to you, rise, pick up your mat, and go home." He rose, picked up his mat at once, and went away in the sight of everyone. They were all astounded and glorified God, saying, "We have never seen anything like this."

So Jesus healed in diverse ways when He walked the earth, and He still, today, heals just as surely. As a matter of fact, His healing power has spread throughout the world through His Church. The Church and Jesus are absolutely inseparable. Jesus never acts without the Church, and the Church can never act effectively without Jesus.

We see in the Acts of the Apostles at the very beginning of the Church, after Jesus had ascended into heaven, that healings continued. These healings were always effected through His Church, however. Could Jesus heal directly in some other way? Most certainly, because He is God. He can do anything and everything in any way He desires. However, He has chosen to act through His Church.

> Many signs and wonders were done among the people at the hands of the apostles. They were together in Solomon's portico. None of the others dared to join him, but the people esteemed them. Yet more than ever, believers of the Lord, great numbers of men and women, were added to

them. Thus they even carried the sick out into the streets and laid them on cots and mats so that when Peter came by, at least his shadow might fall on one or another of them.

Acts 5:12-15

We see that Jesus healed through Peter, the first Pope, the Head of His Church, and through the apostles in union with him. "A large number of people from the towns in the vicinity of Jerusalem also gathered, bringing the sick and those disturbed by unclean spirits, and they were all cured" (Acts 5:16).

So, yes, Christ can heal us physically today. Will He do so? Most certainly and effortlessly, but only if for our overall long term good, that is our eternal salvation and the salvation of others. For He heals in diverse ways including physically and spiritually. He can accomplish physical healings instantaneously and miraculously, outside the laws of nature, or through the means of medical personnel and science, the laws and benefits of which were are all created by Him. His will in regard to our physical healing can be accomplished immediately, quickly, or over many years; or His will may be brought about in our death. As difficult as it is to embrace on a human level, may we believe God's Word when He tells us: "We know that all things work for good for those who love God, who are called according to his purpose" (Romans 8:28).

As I said, illness such as cancer is a figure of a soul sick in sin. We all suffer from the cancer of sin. As cancer attacks, affects, and harms the entire body, so does sin to the Mystical Body of Jesus Christ, of whom we are all directly or implicitly members. "Can it be that the sin of one man (Adam) can have greater effects and disorder in human nature than the Incarnation of the Son of God has in ordering all humanity? That is why I say that everybody in the world is implicitly Christian."[17]

The only *healing balm* for the cancer of sin is Jesus. We bring our cancerous sin to Jesus in contrition, He touches us, and we are healed.

"When Jesus came down from the mountain, great crowds followed him. And then a leper approached, did him homage, and said, 'Lord, if you wish, you can make me clean.'" Cancer, like leprosy, is a strong representation of sin. "He stretched out his hand, touched him, and said, 'I will do it. Be made clean.' His leprosy was cleansed immediately" (Matthew 8:1–3).

What rapture there is in the touch of Jesus!

Jesus's touch is there for each of us for the asking any and every time we seek it or, shall we say, accept it. As I make these analogies, it is important to state that I am not denying the reality of the physical illnesses and healings recorded in Scripture. These miracles truly occurred. I am simply commenting on a more profound spiritual meaning represented in the Word of God, which is infinite in its depth and meaning. We can never exhaust the meaning of Scripture.

I am not an expert on the following; however, I have heard the theory that there are cancer cells that occur in every person's body during the course of his lifetime. These are normally kept in check by a person's healthy immune system. *Jesus is our healthy immune system.* Without Him we would be ravaged very quickly by the cancer of temptation and sin. Jesus acts through the Sacraments of His Church, for example, through Baptism; and through His Body, Blood, Soul, and Divinity in the Eucharist; and through the Sacrament of Reconciliation (also called Penance or Confession). He also keeps us healthy through our prayer which is, or at least should be, the very fresh air for the soul and spirit that we breathe at every moment.

It is good to come to Jesus for His mercy often so that we can kill off the minor vestiges of the cancer of sin that are trying to gain a hold on us. The medicine of Jesus's Body, Blood, Soul, and Divinity, which we Catholics receive in Holy Communion, is the medicine that transforms and incorporates our body, blood, soul, and spirit into our infinitely healthy and holy Jesus Christ, our Lord and Savior. Then, through no merit of our own, our Heavenly Father sees Jesus when He looks at us, and He is well pleased. "And a voice came from the heavens, saying, 'This is my beloved Son, with whom I am well pleased'" (Matthew 3:17).

Jesus, our Lord, is the *ultimate chemotherapy* for the cancer of sin. In an encounter in the Confessional, or in the extraordinary way of a heartfelt, perfect contrition for sins, Christ pours out the always and completely curative chemotherapy of His mercy; and the cancer of sin is obliterated instantaneously and completely. We are covered by His blood through which we have remission of sins. His very perfect and healthy blood courses through our veins reaching every hidden room in our soul, washing everything clean. Nothing is left with the slightest stain.

I was recently blessed to witness my daughter Brighde, age six, come out of the Confessional with a huge smile, pumping her fists in the air, saying "Yes!" (She had special permission from our pastor to receive her first confession at the early age of six.) What joy she exuded knowing that any sins were washed away by the Precious Blood of Jesus through His priest. We can learn so much from the innocence and simplicity of children. I, for one, am going to try to learn from Brighde's example of appreciating this sublime sacrament more. One can never value the Sacrament of Reconciliation (Confession) enough, as it cost the blood and death of our Lord Jesus to give it to us.

And God will often use modern medicine to effect our physical cure. God often works through our wonderful, dedicated, compassionate, medical personnel (this has been my experience). What a noble profession! Science, including medicine, should not decrease our faith in God. It ought to increase our faith, for all things are created by Him. He gave us everything on earth to develop for our use, and for our good. "God created man in his image;/ in the divine image he created him; 'male and female he created them'. God blessed them, saying to them: 'Be fertile and multiply; fill the earth and subdue it....God looked at everything he had made, and he found it very good'" (Genesis 1:27–31).

As for God working through modern medicine, we turn to Sirach 38:1–15:

> Hold the physician in honor, for he is essential to you,/ and God it was who established his profession./ From God the doctor has his wisdom,/ and the king provides for his sustenance./ His knowledge makes the doctor distinguished,/ and gives him access to those in authority./ God makes the earth yield healing herbs/ which the prudent man should not neglect;/ Was not the water sweetened by a twig/ that men might learn his power?/ He endows men with the knowledge/ to glory in his mighty works,/ Through which the doctor eases pain/ and the druggist prepares his medicines;/ Thus God's creative work continues without cease/ in its efficacy on the surface of the earth./
>
> My son, when you are ill, delay not,/ but pray to God, who will heal you:/ Flee wickedness; let your hands be just,/ cleanse your heart of every sin;/ Offer your sweet-smelling oblation and petition,/ a rich offering according to your means./ Then give the doctor his place/ lest he leave; for you need him too./ There are times that give him an advantage,/ and he too beseeches God/ That his diagnosis may be correct/ and his treatment bring about a cure./ He who is a sinner toward his Maker/ will be defiant toward the doctor.

So modern medicine is good and should be utilized, but mixed with our prayers, almsgiving, and avoidance and cleansing of sin, out of love of God.

On November 12, 2010, I noticed the beginning of a rash on my belly and inner thigh. The rash was mild that day when I saw my oncologist. We suspected a drug reaction to Moxiofloxacin, an antibiotic I had been taking for sixteen days to treat pneumonia (a side effect of my leukemia and treatment, both having a significant effect on reducing my immune system). We decided to discontinue the antibiotic. By Saturday, November 13, the rash was twenty times worse. I also developed a fever and increased pulse. The doctor on call at Northwestern Hospital suggested that I go to the emergency room that evening. In the course of the evening my temperature went over 103 degrees. I was admitted to the hospital once again, the sixth time in approximately one year.

My fever was quickly brought under control, but the rash became enormously worse. The rash had spread from my feet to the top of my head. Eventually the only part of my body spared were the palms of my hands and the soles of my feet.

The rash ended up covering my body almost completely with little or no unaffected skin surface. My entire body turned red with the lower extremities turning especially bright red thanks to a combination, apparently, of the rash and low platelets, wherein I was bleeding into the skin.

Various teams of doctors came into my room including both the regular team on the floor and an infectious disease team and dermatology team. The rash also developed blisters. I felt and apparently looked very much like Job who was struck from head to toe with something that sounds similar. "So Satan went forth from the presence of the LORD and smote Job with severe boils from the soles of his feet to the crown of his head. And he took a potsherd to scrape himself, as he sat among the ashes" (Job 2:7–8).

I was quarantined. The medical teams had to cover their bases and came up with various theories on what might be the cause of my rash. A number of the doctors referred to my rash as very "impressive." What an interesting compliment. Just what I always wanted—to impress people with my rash. The infectious disease and dermatology team requested permission to take pictures of the rash, which I agreed to. One doctor nonchalantly told me that it might be a certain virus, in which case I might die. I think he trained medical personnel in bedside manner... not! (Overall the doctors and medical personnel at Northwestern were overwhelmingly great, talented, and very empathetic. I am especially grateful to my hematologists/oncologists and to the doctor who oversaw my stem-cell transplant. I cannot say enough good about them. I am exceedingly grateful to them all.)

Next, all of my important blood counts plummeted, including white counts, but especially my platelets, which dropped very rapidly from 99,000 on November 12 down to 12,000 on November 17. Once they drop under 10,000, a transfusion is generally needed as there is a risk of spontaneous internal bleeding which could lead to death. The situation appeared bleak. My rash had eventually turned purple and looked like it would take an awfully long time to heal.

During this time in the hospital I was really not feeling very bad physically. I kept up exercise and most especially my prayer life. I prayed the rosary and, as always, turned to Scripture. I opened my Bible spontaneously to numerous encouraging passages, many of which I include in the chapter "Healing Scripture Passages" for the encouragement, fortitude, and consolation of the reader. I include a few here as well.

"'Though alive, I am among the dead. I can hear a man's voice, but I cannot see him.' Raphael said, 'Take courage! God has healing in store for you; so take courage!'" (Tobit 5:10).

"You shall find your tent secure, and your sheepfold untouched when you come. You shall see your descendants multiply, your offspring grow like the grass in the fields. In ripe old age you shall go to the grave" (Job 5:24–26, JB).

"It is the LORD who marches before you; he will be with you and will never fail you or forsake you. So do not fear or be dismayed" (Deuteronomy 31:8).

My prayer gave me great hope. One cannot have an infallible knowledge that he will recover, but I certainly had a sense and encouragement in my prayer that I would. It also needs to be said that there were numerous people praying for me, as usual. Thanks be to God and to these generous souls.

On approximately November 18 my rash began to rapidly get better. What seemed to be the impossible happened very quickly. In a matter of just a few days the rash was almost completely gone except for on my lower legs. As a matter of fact, I was released from the hospital on Saturday November 20, and within another couple of days the rash was essentially gone with the exception of a handful of blisters still finishing to heal. I do not see how anyone can deny God's hand in this rapid recovery.

My platelets, which had dropped to 12,000 on November 17, took a turn up later in the day to 19,000. By November 18 they were up to 37,000. By November 22 they were up to 128,000. This was with no medical intervention. What was confirmed as a drug reaction to the Moxiofloxacin had apparently run its course, allowing for the healing; however, the speed of the recovery leads me to give glory to God, the "author of saving acts" (Psalms 74:12, JB).

I continue to trust my infinitely loving Father in heaven who is seeing to everything for my good. I know that nothing can happen to me or touch me unless He says so. His timing and providence in our lives is perfect. "There is nothing to fear. Everyone moved by the Spirit is a son of God. The spirit you received is not the spirit of slaves bringing fear into your lives again; it is the spirit of sons, and it makes us cry out, 'Abba, Father!'" (Romans 8:14–16, JB).

Do I always live this level of trust and faith? No, but I am quickly reinvigorated when I turn to prayer and the Sacraments. Praised be Jesus! Thank You, Heavenly Father, for everything! Thank You for being my faithful Father!

HEALING IN MIND

"But the Lord answered: 'Martha, Martha,' he said 'you worry and fret about so many things, and yet few are needed, indeed only one. It is Mary who has chosen the better part; it is not to be taken from her'" (Luke 10:41–42, JB).

In this passage we find Martha's sister, Mary, sitting at the feet of Jesus while Martha is doing all the fretting and serving. Our human activities can be necessary, but few are needed; and they are always inferior to God. Jesus is the *Better Part*. Jesus is telling us that we will only find peace if choose the Better Part, by placing Him as number one in our lives.

Worry comes easily to me as I imagine it does to many. We do tend to worry and fret about many things. I am well aware that I am only sustained by the constant help of God. As long as I don't rebel, which I unfortunately do to my own detriment many times, I am fine. Thank God for the Sacrament of Penance, also known as "Confession," to help me back on my feet. It is only when I choose to push God aside that I get into trouble.

Many worries crossed my mind after my diagnosis. How will my family be provided for if I die? How will my wife, Kathleen, manage the family without me? Though Kathleen is a wonderful, faith-filled leader, she needs my help; how will she keep our children on the narrow road of faith and virtue in this challenging culture? How will my family be protected? How will my work of evangelization be accomplished? What will become of my small business? The answer to these questions, fears, and doubts, as always, was to *trust in Jesus.*

It is easy to trust in Him when everything is going our way, but the pedal meets the metal when we receive a challenging cross like cancer in our lives. As I prayed about this, I came to the hard-to-accept, yet encouraging and true, reminder that God does not need me to accomplish any of these things. Don't misunderstand—we each have a mission and responsibilities that God has given us to fulfill, and we must do our best to accomplish them, but only for as long as God decides. Our irreplaceable mission in life can only be achieved by ourselves—no one else; so we do have a serious obligation to put our talents to work for God's glory while we have the gift of life here on earth.

I am currently gifted with the privilege of leading and serving my family. God most certainly has the power to take care of my family in His special, mysterious, and providential way even better without me, if He so chooses. I know that whatever He chooses will be the best. I do want to go on living to care for my family and enjoy the beautiful gift of life, but this is outside of my control. It is in God's control! He can accomplish the work of caring for my family and evangelization without me. My only responsibility is to be true to my call to work at my mission while I am alive and able. That is my piece of His puzzle. Others have their piece. They will complete their part of the puzzle with their mission and work. After all, "it is all God's work" (2 Corinthians 5:18, JB).

So the answer is to abandon myself into God's trustworthy hands, to embrace God's most perfect plan for me and my family, with confidence and trust that all will work out for the best. Sometimes, on a human level, I am tempted to tell God that my family needs me, so please heal me ASAP. But I then need to, and do, return to the prayer "Father…if you are willing, take this cup away from me. Nevertheless, let your will be done, not mine" (Luke 22:42–43, JB). You, God, are all-knowing and know best, not me. We will only find peace when we abandon ourselves with complete trust into the loving arms of our caring Father.

I have a concrete model to emulate in my children, especially the younger ones. For example, Mairead, age nine; Brighde, age six; and Shealagh, age five, never have a worry. True, they may become momentarily upset about something, but they quickly regain their peace and joy. They never worry about where their next meal is coming from, or about having a roof over their heads, about their health, how the bills will be paid, or about how they will pay for college over a decade down the road. If they get a "booboo," Daddy takes care of it.

They are more about being than having, grasping, and controlling. Place them outside with no toys, and they quickly invent toys with small tree branches, or are engaged in a game they promptly put together. They can often be observed carelessly and joyfully running around merrily. With a little reflection one can easily see the wisdom and truth in this Scripture passage: "Jesus, however, called the children to himself and said, 'Let the children come to me and do not prevent them; for the kingdom of God belongs to such as these'" (Luke 18:16).

I recall from my diary an example of the innocence and innate spirituality of little children in an occurrence involving my daughter Shealagh when she was three years of age. "December 2, 2009: Today she was transfigured, happy, kissing and hugging me. She told me at Mass, 'Jesus loves me when I love you.' I told her that Jesus always loves her."

Another memory involving my daughter Brighde, at age five, gleaned from my diary.

> February 16, 2010: Yesterday I received the skull cap of Venerable, Archbishop Fulton J. Sheen, from [a friend]. It is on loan for a couple of days. As soon as I received it and opened the box containing it, Brighde, Fulton J. Sheen's goddaughter, came up to me, not knowing what I had, and

out of the blue began reciting the poem/prayer "Lovely Lady Dressed in Blue," which happens to be a favorite of Archbishop Fulton J. Sheen. Brighde did this without any prompting. This was a beautiful grace. The Archbishop is definitely interceding from heaven.

I will often compliment Brighde and Shealagh saying, "You are the most beautiful girl in the world", or, "You are so wonderful, smart, and good." They will respectively answer in simplicity something to the effect, "I know." Young children accept so naturally the truth that they are loved and are loveable, and they naturally love in return. Have we forgotten how loveable we truly are? "We have come to know and to believe in the love God has for us" (1 John 4:16).

To God, your Father, each of you is the most beautiful person in the world, despite your human faults. As a matter of fact, our faults make us even more loveable, analogous to how we see our young children when they make a mistake. We should accept this. I love my children beyond measure, but believe me, God our Father loves each of us infinitely more than whatever human love we can muster.

Sometimes in their innocence and inherent good my children will say to me: "You're the best daddy." Of course, I am not the best daddy, which gives me cause to want to work harder to truly be a better dad, though I appreciate the love behind the compliment. But be assured that God our Father is the best Dad. Wouldn't it be a beautiful prayer to simply tell Him: "You're the best Daddy!" A good dad does not spare his child every challenge in life, but encourages him or her through the tests so that the child might grow in strength, virtue, maturity, etc. Can we expect less from our perfect Father in heaven as we grow and progress toward our heavenly homeland?

Has your father or someone very close to you ever said, "I would do anything for you?" This is only a dim reflection of the sentiments and action of our Father in heaven, and He always means and does what He says. He would do anything for us, and He has already given us His very best in sending His only Son to die on the cross, and rise from the dead, to save us.

Children are eminently trusting souls. By the time my children are in late high school or college, they begin to worry about the future—things like education, money, and finding the right spouse. What happens to us as we grow older? How do we become so jaded and tending toward anxiety? I believe it is part of the cross of our human nature that each of us is called to bear, but this cross, like any cross, becomes a good deal lighter when we permit Jesus to carry the bulk of it for us. He is always there desiring to help us.

Did you ever notice how the elderly often tend to become more like children, dependent on others, trusting others for their sustenance? Loving and trusting in God is the opposite of the fear, worry, and anxiety that we are so prone to as adults.

My father was recently diagnosed with the early stages of Alzheimer's disease. I have seen other relatives go through this. At some advanced point they became very similar to babies in that they depended on others for everything, including eating and going to the bathroom. Society may see little value in their lives, but isn't life worth more than the current quality of one's intellect, the ability to communicate well, or how productive that person may be? In God's eyes a baby or an advanced Alzheimer's patient is just as valuable as the smartest, most productive adult!

We are wonderfully made in the image and likeness of God. "I thank you: for the wonder of myself, for the wonder of your works. You know me through and through" (Psalm 139:14, JB). And God knows and loves us, without measure, better than anyone else does.

God does not value us for our strengths. As a matter of fact, He values us most for our weakness. "My grace is enough for you: my power is at its best in weakness" (2 Corinthians 12:9, JB). Every stage of life from conception, when the egg is fertilized, until the last moment of natural death is sacred, a gift from God, that should never be tampered with.

How much our minds today are scattered, busy, overloaded, and hurting! Add to this the many worries of everyday life including health, family, and work. Our minds need healing. We need peace.

Cancer and other serious crosses can help us to put our priorities in order. We need to take time out to rest our minds, and to contemplate the reality that the things of this world are passing. Most of us regularly need to slow down, come to a deserted place, turn off our televisions, computers, smartphones, etc., and rest a while. Jesus has directed us so. "He said to them, 'Come away by yourselves to a deserted place and rest a while.' People were coming and going in great numbers, and they had no opportunity even to eat" (Mark 6:31).

It is important for us to keep in mind the unconditional fact that Jesus is with us. "And know that I am with you always: yes, to the end of time" (Matthew 28:20, JB). He loves us, and we love Him; He is "turning everything to their good" (Romans 8:28, JB). If one does not love God, He needs to ask God, the Source of all love, to fill Him with His love that he might love Him back. This prayer will always be answered in the affirmative. "How much more will your Father in heaven give good things to those who ask him!" (Matthew 7:11, JB).

We can truly walk through life without a care if we have a great faith and peace, which is a gift available for the asking. "If God is for us, who can be against us?" (Romans 8:31). Of course, our human nature will often rebel, as does mine, but deep down we will have peace because we know that our Father is God, and He always cares for His children! "As a father has compassion on his children,/ so the LORD has compassion on the faithful" (Psalm 103:13).

We tend to worry too much and unnecessarily. So many of us bring a great deal of needless anxiety down upon ourselves by worrying about the future, often twenty or more years ahead. For example: "If I have another child, how will I afford college for him or her eighteen years down the road?" One can plan prudently but never be strictly in control of the outcome. We need to remember that God is in supreme control. That is not negotiable. He is driving the car, and He is good at it, much better than we are. We are called to exercise our free will to trust Him. We need to stop grabbing the steering wheel from Him. He is in the driver's seat. We can let our minds rest and even take a refreshing nap on His shoulder while He is at the wheel.

Jesus only gave us permission to be concerned about today, not tomorrow. "So do not worry about tomorrow: tomorrow will take care of itself. Each day has enough trouble of its own" (Matthew 6:34, JB). Jesus understands our limited capacity: "he knows what we are made of" (Psalm 103:14, JB). As a matter of fact, He himself makes up for our limitations in every conceivable way, including dying on the cross for us out of infinite love to save us from our sins when we could not save ourselves. His loving providence is always at work for our good and the good of others.

We are not designed—we do not have the capacity, being only human—to carry the extra weight of worries about the future which are outside of our control. This also applies to cancer. Will this cancer kill me? Will my treatment work? Other than doing what we can to take care of the gift of our health, like good nutrition, proper rest, exercise, and pursuing proper medical care, the rest is ultimately out of our control. We cannot know what will happen to us tomorrow let alone a year from now.

It usually turns out that the things we worry most about never come to pass, or work out differently, quite often for the better, than what we worked ourselves up about. If they do happen, they are not nearly as bad as we had dreaded, and we may be given a glimpse into the Wisdom to see the good that came out of the difficulty.

Rather than exhausting and tormenting ourselves with worry and anxiety, we can use that energy for what is truly important in our lives, to live by a hierarchy of values—foremost God, then family, then friends, and then work and service to others, in that order of importance. We become happier this way, closer to living the way God designed us to live. True, this is impossible to our human nature alone. That is why we need and must seek and accept God's help, always readily available to us.

"Do not give in to sadness,/ torment not yourself with brooding; Gladness of heart is the very life of man,/ cheerfulness prolongs his days./ Distract yourself, renew your courage,/ drive resentment far away from you;/ For worry has brought death to many,/ nor is there aught to be gained from resentment" (Sirach 30:21–23). What can we gain by worry and sadness but additions to our suffering? Why be resentful or brood over getting cancer or that others don't seem to care or help us enough according to our self-centered outlook? We are not in control. God is! He is God. We are not. Thanks be to God that He is in charge, because left completely to ourselves we would encounter disaster.

We are called to be cheerful, because we have God on our side. When we make an effort to smile and be cheerful, we tend to actually become happier. We need courage to live all this, which comes from God.

> For what man knows God's counsel,/ or who can conceive what our LORD intends?/ For the deliberations of mortals are timid,/ and unsure are our plans./ For the corruptible body burdens the soul/ and the earthen shelter weighs down the mind that has many concerns./ And scarce do we guess the things on earth,/ and what is within our grasp we find with difficulty;/ but when things are in heaven, who can search them out?/ Or who ever knew your counsel, except you had given Wisdom/ and sent your holy spirit from on high?/ And thus were the paths of those on earth

made straight,/ and men learned what was your pleasure,/ and were saved by Wisdom.

Wisdom 9:13–18

Yes, only the Holy Spirit can give us true wisdom! We need to dump out our self-centeredness so God can fill us with Himself.

My son, why increase your cares,/ since he who is avid for wealth will not be blameless?/ Even if you run after it, you will never overtake it;/ however you seek it, you will not find it./ One may toil and struggle and drive,/ and fall short all the more./ Another goes his way a weakling and a failure,/ with little strength and great misery—/Yet the eyes of the LORD look favorably upon him;/ he raises him free of the vile dust,/ Lifts up his head and exalts him/ to the amazement of the many./ Good and evil, life and death,/ poverty and riches, are from the LORD./ Wisdom and understanding and knowledge of affairs,/ love and virtuous paths are from the LORD./ Error and darkness were formed with sinners from their birth,/ and evil grows old with evildoers./ The LORD's gift remains with the just;/ his favor brings continued success.

Sirach 11:10–17

Yes, everything good comes from God. And it is good to focus on our blessings more than the things that do not go our way. Lord, You have given me another day, my faith in You, my breath, a wonderful wife, a beautiful family, friends, the splendor of nature, some work or activity to engage in, my daily sustenance…. Thank You for being so generous to me, Father.

"A blessing on the man who puts his trust in Yahweh, with Yahweh for his hope. He is like a tree by the waterside that thrusts its roots to the stream: when the heat comes it feels no alarm, its foliage stays green; it has no worries in a year of drought, and never ceases to bear fruit" (Jeremiah 17:7–8, JB). When we trust in God like little children, His Kingdom belongs to us! There are no worries.

I visited Melbourne, Australia, several years ago, to help in my small way promote vocations to the priesthood and consecrated life in the Catholic Church. I really liked the phrase that was often used among the Australians: *No worries*. We, beyond doubt, have no worries when we have God. We are confident that our lives are continuing to bear fruit even when the years of drought, such as cancer, assail us. What drought in history did not eventually pass?

> Rejoice in the Lord always. I shall say it again: rejoice! Your kindness should be known to all. The Lord is near. Have no anxiety at all, but in everything, by prayer and petition, with thanksgiving, make your requests known to God. Then the peace of God that surpasses all understanding will guard your hearts and minds in Christ Jesus.
>
> Finally, brothers, whatever is true, whatever is honorable, whatever is just, whatever is pure, whatever is lovely, whatever is gracious, if there is any excellence and if there is anything worthy of praise, think about these things.
>
> Philippians 4:4–8

God tells us to have no anxiety about anything. He makes no exceptions. Neither should we. When we live the way God intends for us, we will be happy and at peace. All we have to do is to let God know what we need, with thanksgiving, and we can leave everything confidently in His hands to do what is best for us every time. Though He already knows what we need, He wants us to exercise our faith and free will by humbly asking, acknowledging our limitations and His omnipotence and generosity.

We can then be at peace, the real peace that surpasses all understanding, knowing that all is in His good hands. Especially with a cross like cancer, which is ultimately out of our control, it is liberating to give it to God completely with a childlike trust, and leave the worry to Him to be obliterated.

We can help to receive and apply God's gift of peace by using our God-given faculties to think positively, to think about good and virtuous things: *think about these things*.

HEALING THROUGH TRUST AND SURRENDER

"Be still and confess that I am God!" (Psalm 46:11).
Some edited excerpts from my diary:

January 25, 2011, Conversion of St. Paul: Today I am being admitted to Northwestern Memorial Hospital for my stem-cell transplant. My recent bone marrow biopsy revealed that there are still 50 percent leukemia/cancer cells in the bone marrow. Therefore, I will need the intermediate-level conditioning chemotherapy, the more intensive of the two the medical team was considering for me. I am ready by the grace of God. This is a gift.

January 26, 2011, St. Timothy and Titus, Bishops and January 27, 2011, St. Angela Merici, Virgin: I have received heavy-duty therapy for these two days, which I seem to tolerate fairly well. I feel strong, by the grace of God. Part of the process was heavy hydration via IV fluids that caused me to quickly gain about 8 pounds and suffer some edema in my ankles and feet.

This was quickly overcome by the morning of January 28.

January 28, 2011, St. Thomas Aquinas, Priest and Doctor of the Church: Today is my "birthday" in which I will receive my generous donor's stem cells. (He currently remains anonymous, but is apparently international.) These stem cells will hopefully overcome the cancer and leave me with a new, healthy immune system, if God so wills it.

In my morning meditation today, among many other encouraging passages I encountered in my Bible, I came upon Romans 15:4–6 (JB): "And indeed everything that was written long ago in the Scriptures was meant to teach us something about hope from the examples Scripture gives of how people who did not give up were helped by God. And may he who helps us when we refuse to give up, help you all to be tolerant with each other, following the example of Christ Jesus, so that united in mind and voice you may give glory to the God and Father of our Lord Jesus Christ."

Today, being the Memorial of St. Thomas Aquinas in the Catholic Church, encourages me to continue working to complete this book. St. Thomas Aquinas was a prolific writer. This morning there was a beautiful sunrise, the first day the sun has shone since I was admitted to the hospital. I have been gifted with an awesome room. Two entire walls are windows overlooking downtown Chicago and Lake Michigan from the fifteenth floor. I am sure our Blessed Mother Mary was behind interceding with Jesus to obtain this tremendous hospital room for us.

I am blessed beyond words to have my beautiful bride, Kathleen, accompanying me every moment, day and night, through this journey in the hospital. This is true sacrificial love on her part. [She actually stayed with me for the entire four-week stay, day and night, sleeping in my hospital room, only returning home for two nights to be with our children, who also visited often.] I am grateful to my adult children for coming together to watch our large family while Kathleen and I are away.

This morning the first reading for the Mass is quintessentially apropos to Kathleen and I—Hebrews 10:32–39: "Remember the days past when, after you had been enlightened, you endured a great contest of suffering. At times you were publicly exposed to abuse and affliction; at other times you associated yourselves with those so treated. You even joined in the sufferings of those in prison and joyfully accepted the confiscation of your property while knowing you had a better and lasting possession. Therefore do not throw away your confidence; it will have great recompense. You need endurance to do the will of God and receive what he has promised./ For after just a brief moment,/ he who is to come shall come;/ he shall not delay./ But my just one shall live by faith,/ and if he draws back I take no pleasure in him./ We are not among those who draw back and perish but among those who have faith and will possess life" (Lectionary for the Mass).

January 29, 2011 St. Gildas, the Wise, Abbot: I have been blessed with some beautiful consolations in my prayer this morning. I know that God is with me. "Yahweh Sabaoth, happy the man who puts his trust in you!" (Psalm 84:12, JB).

"I know the plans I have in mind for you—it is Yahweh who speaks—plans for peace, not disaster, reserving a future full of hope for you" (Jeremiah 29:11–12, JB).

January 30, 2011: Today I broke out in an apparently drug-related rash. In addition to the rash, I have diarrhea. God is with us. Jesus, I trust in You! I have placed everything in our Blessed Mother Mary's hands with confidence.

January 31, 2011, St. John Bosco: This morning in my mediation I received many lights of encouragement. I opened my Bible at random: "'Lord, the man you love is ill.'

121

On receiving the message, Jesus said, 'This sickness will end not in death but in God's glory, and through it the Son of God will be glorified'" (John 11:4, JB).

February 1, 2011: This evening I am suffering extreme fatigue, nausea, and unfounded anxiety. All for Jesus and souls!

February 2, 2011: Feast of the Presentation: Last night I was unable to sleep for the better part of the night suffering anxiety, with my mind racing uncontrollably. This morning I learned that I am now neutropenic, meaning that I have no measurable white cells left to fight infection. This is part of the stem-cell transplant process to be expected; however, the risk of infection is at its height. All for Jesus and souls!

The Feast of the Presentation commemorates the day Joseph and Mary presented Jesus at the temple forty days after His birth. This is also the Feast in the Catholic Church that supports, honors, and promotes religious and consecrated men and women. It is interesting that during the night or perhaps the early morning hours I was thinking that my daughter Colleen, who is a consecrated woman in the Church, was in the room with me. I prayed for her and offered my sufferings for her, and also for my son Shane, who is discerning and studying for the priesthood. Jesus, Mary, and St. Joseph, we love you, save souls. St. Simeon, pray for us. St. Anna, pray for us.

Yesterday afternoon, all night, and this morning there was a major snowstorm, the snowstorm of 2011, third biggest in the history of Chicago! We had an interesting bird's eye view from the fifteenth floor of the hospital. Many major roads were closed, etc.

Last night during my suffering I turned to Jesus, "meek and humble of heart" (Matthew 11:29), whose *yolk is easy and burden light* (see Matthew 11:30), and I asked to place my head on His breast, that He might relieve me of some of the suffering I am experiencing, if it be His most holy will. Later this morning, Father Bill, the hospital chaplain, visited me, and in his counsel after my confession (I can talk about it, though he can't) he said that I should give my cross to Jesus to carry and to let Him embrace me. This is in line with my prayers during the night. Thanks be to God for people and priests like Father Bill. He is always speaking of Jesus's love for us, and our need to surrender to it, to accept it, to know that He forgives us all our failings (when we are truly contrite).

As my four-week stay for the stem-cell transplant progressed, I experienced some major setbacks. I ended up in ICU with total kidney failure resulting in the need for dialysis. They had to insert a central line in my jugular vein for the dialysis in spite of my platelets being at 3,000. Normal starts at 150,000. Platelets help the blood to clot. The medical personnel were afraid I would bleed to death during the insertion. It took a brave doctor to attempt the procedure. I also had double fungal pneumonia.

My heart was racing at a sustained rate of 200 beats per minute. My blood pressure was extremely high. I could hardly speak, and then, with a great effort, only in a sort of hoarse whisper. At one point I was so sick that I had no energy left to fight. I think I still had fight in my soul and will with the assistance of the Holy Spirit, but my body was extremely sick and feeble. I exchanged what seemed to be our final words with my wife, Kathleen, basically expressing our love between us, my wishes about our family, and saying good-bye until heaven.

On top of my health challenges our personal checking account was garnished and frozen by a creditor during this hospital stay.

It was intriguing that, shortly after I was wheeled into my intensive-care room, a Catholic priest appeared in my room. Kathleen tells me that this was at about 10:00 p.m. on Super Bowl Sunday. It turns out that he had stepped into my room to get out of the way while waiting to see another patient in ICU. What are the odds of a Catholic priest coming into my room at a pivotal life-and-death moment like this, at a time like this? I admit that this made me think that I was likely going to die, as God had arranged for this priest to be there to pave my way into eternity. I asked him for the Sacraments of Penance (Confession) and the Anointing of the Sick, which he readily administered. I was cleansed of all sin, ready for eternity. I had already received Jesus in Holy Communion earlier in the day. As a matter of fact, I had never missed a day receiving Holy Communion during my hospital stays, as Kathleen, my older daughters, Shannon and Tara, and various ministers at the hospital brought me Jesus daily. Thanks be to God, I was proven wrong about my expectation of possibly dying at that time. It shows that only God knows the hour when He will call us. He is in command, thanks be to Him.

I had some intense spiritual experiences in the ICU. I believed I was dying. I learned even more clearly the power of intercessory prayer. God has given each of us a share in His power to help others as well as ourselves with our prayers and suffering. Prayer is the most powerful means we have been gifted with.

By the grace of God, I was saved again. I progressively recovered to the point of being released from ICU. When I was returned to my regular room in the hospital it seemed impossible to walk due to being in bed so long and all that I had gone through. However, the first day back to my room I did get up and walk with a walker. One of the medical personnel commented that she had never seen anyone get out of bed as quick as me after being in ICU; all the glory to God.

My body had swollen up with fluids. My abdomen was distended and hard. I had gone from my weight of 195 pounds when entering the hospital to 236 pounds. I had atrophied about twenty pounds, which means I had approximately 60 pounds of toxic fluid to eliminate from my body. Dialysis helped with this, and my kidneys began functioning a bit so that I could urinate quite often. My weight eventually went down to 175 pounds with all the fluids washed out. God is truly the "author of saving acts" (Psalm 74:12, JB).

Eventually my blood counts began to rise indicating that the donor cells were engrafting. If the stem-cell transplant is successful, it takes about six to twelve months to recover substantially, and three years or so to recover fully.

After four weeks in the hospital I was released to home, where I quickly graduated from the walker to a cane to walking without a cane, and where I gradually regained my strength to where I was taking long walks, jogging short distances, playing basketball with my children, though very poorly, and climbing three hundred steps up a stairway on a sand dune, thanks be to God. "There is nothing I cannot master with the help of the One who gives me strength" (Philippians 4:13–14, JB).

After my stem-cell transplant I found that even though I did not feel up to it, the more I forced myself to get up and around and be active, the better I felt, and the more improved my health seemed to become. I tried to work up toward engaging in as much of my normal activity as possible. I found that this activity strengthened, energized, and revitalized me. This not only helped my body, but just as importantly it helped my mind, attitude, and spirit. I am convinced that if I had sat and lain around much of the day, which is what I felt like doing, my recovery time would have been much longer, or I may have regressed. I know that this activity is not always possible for everyone, but where health permits, I believe it is helpful to be as active as possible, of course within reason and with some moderation, though admittedly moderation is not my normal modus operandi.

Let's reflect on Luke 14:25–33.

> Great crowds were traveling with him, and he turned and addressed them, "If any one comes to me without hating his father and mother, wife and children, brothers and sisters,

and even his own life, he cannot be my disciple. Whoever does not carry his own cross and come after me cannot be my disciple."

Jesus is not asking us to literally hate our relatives and our own life. He is inviting us to love them but with detachment so we can put Him first in every way, at all times. As a matter of fact, when we love God above everyone and everything, we are filled by Him with a greater capacity to appreciate the gift of our lives, and to sacrificially love others, the kind of true love that costs us something, like Jesus demonstrated on the cross.

Yes, Jesus is not only asking a lot of us, He is asking everything of us. He wants to be our All, because He knows that this is what we were made for and the only way to fulfillment. This requires carrying the cross, which is very challenging. Getting started in following Christ can sometimes seem easy and full of pleasantries. However, because Jesus loves us so much, He is demanding and will challenge us even beyond what we think we are capable of, although He will never truly challenge us beyond our true capabilities.

> Which of you wishing to construct a tower does not first sit down and calculate the cost to see if there is enough for its completion? Otherwise, after laying the foundation and finding himself unable to finish the work the onlookers should laugh at him and say, "This one began to build but did not have the resources to finish."

> Luke 14:28–30

To construct a tower is a long and challenging process. One enters into such a project with at least the reasonable foreknowledge of the demands and duration of the project. Following Christ is about enduring until the end. It is about finishing. It is the long,

126

hard, narrow, but fruitful road. The prize, the completed tower, is no less than our eternal salvation and the salvation of others whom we help along the way.

> Or what king marching into battle would not first sit down and decide whether with ten thousand troops he can successfully oppose another king advancing upon him with twenty thousand troops? But if not, while he is still far away, he will send a delegation to ask for peace terms. In the same way, everyone of you who does not renounce all his possessions cannot be my disciple.

Luke 14:31–33

I could never understand this passage about the king marching into battle until very recently. I think the Holy Spirit has finally given me a long-awaited insight into its meaning, perhaps so that I can share it with you. As with many things of God, His ways are 180 degrees different than the way we would see or expect things. I believe that, in the ways of God, the king who surrendered and asked for peace terms was truly the winner here. And that surrendering king is you and me.

I believe that Christ is portrayed as the victorious, powerful king advancing with twenty thousand troops. What would the surrendering king in a situation like this have to concede in order to win peace? Probably everything. The victorious king would likely take most if not all of His power and possessions. We, who often see ourselves as, and who act as, kings in control of our own little kingdoms, are called to surrender to the true King, Jesus Christ, who is all powerful, but enormously benevolent. We are wise to sue for peace, the peace that Christ offers us, which can only be obtained by giving Him everything, by making Him our All, by bowing down in reverence and adoration to Him.

But Christ is not like a worldly king who takes advantage of his power and victory and lords it over us.

> You know that those who are recognized as rulers over the Gentiles lord it over them, and their great ones make their authority over them felt. But it shall not be so among you. Rather, whoever wishes to become great among you will be your servant; whoever wishes to be first among you will be the slave of all. For the Son of Man did not come to be served but to serve and to give his life as a ransom for many.
>
> Mark 10:42–45

By surrendering to Christ the King, He gives us victory. He is never outdone in generosity. He gives us infinitely more than what we have surrendered to Him. We give Him our attachments to our little possessions, which we had wanted to remain in control of and sought our security in—such as others, our health, power, materialism, intellect, pursuit of unbridled pleasure—and He gives us the best, Himself, Everything! He gives us His infinite love and mercy. He lays down His life for us! We become His subjects so that He can exalt us, wait on us, and wash our feet. He is the Heavenly King, our eternal God, the Word who humbled Himself and became flesh so that He could save us from our sins and heal us.

> Who, though he was in the form of God,/ did not regard equality with God/ something to be grasped./ Rather, he emptied himself,/ taking the form of a slave,/ coming in human likeness;/ and found human in appearance,/ he humbled himself,/ becoming obedient to death,/ even death on a cross.
>
> Philippians 2:6–8

He is the type of king who in turn at our Baptism anoints each of us priest, prophet, and king. He gives us His mother, Mary, as our Queen, the Queen of all the angels and saints, to intercede on our behalf and make sure we do not become lost along the way. She always leads us to Jesus, her Son, so we will follow Him because we are nothing without Him; we have no wine. "When the wine ran short, the mother of Jesus said to him, 'They have no wine.' (And) Jesus said to her, 'Woman, how does your concern affect me? My hour has not yet come.' His mother said to the servers, 'Do whatever he tells you'" (John 2:3–5).

Everything in this world is passing. We are made for God, to love and be loved by God in community with our brothers and sisters, and to be perfectly happy for all eternity. Please God, do not let my free will and my pride stand in the way of my daily surrender—no, my surrender every second—to You. Help me, Lord, to love You and to love my neighbor, and to never put inferior things ahead of You, my King. Although everything You created is good, everything is inferior to You, because they are not You. Thank You for showing us Your hands and Your side, and conferring Your peace on us, the only true peace, for You are the King of Peace. "Jesus came and stood in their midst and said to them, 'Peace be with you.' When he had said this, he showed them his hands and his side. The disciples rejoiced when they saw the Lord" (John 20:19–20).

The peace that Jesus offers to us is a divine, heavenly peace which takes root in the superior part of our souls, if only we turn to Him in prayer and accept it, the gift that it is. He loves each of us so incredibly much and desires to shower graces upon us. "Peace I leave with you; my peace I give to you. Not as the world gives do I give it to you. Do not let your hearts be troubled or afraid" (John 14:27).

God provides all that we truly need. He knows what is best for each of us better than we do about ourselves.

Yet I concede that it is very difficult to suffer. It is not easy for me. I want to recommend something to you. Keep saying, "Jesus, I trust in You!" Give everything over to Him and rest your mind and spirit. Rest in the most intimate Sacred Heart of Jesus, from which all of His love, purity, and divine virtues spring forth to us. Abandon yourself to Him, and rest. Put your feet up, "to live there [in His Sacred Heart] and never leave it; to live in purity as bees in the chalice of a lily."[18] He will never *hand you a stone when you ask for a loaf of bread* (see Matthew 7:9). In Him you will always find peace. This kind of trust may be hard to muster, so ask Him for this special grace. The battle is His. Give it over to Him.

There is a 100 percent chance of everything working out for the best in our Merciful Father's plan, as He is always bringing about a tremendous good. "We know that by turning everything to their good God co-operates with all those who love him, with all those that he has called according to his purpose" (Romans 8:28, JB).

> The LORD says to you: "Do not fear or lose heart at the sight of this vast multitude, for the battle is not yours but God's. Go down against them tomorrow....You will not have to fight in this encounter. Take your places, stand firm, and see how the LORD will be with you to deliver you, Judah and Jerusalem. Do not fear or lose heart. Tomorrow go out to meet them, and the LORD will be with you..."
>
> "Trust in the LORD, your God, and you will be found firm."
>
> 2 Chronicles 20:15–20

In Scripture God is constantly encouraging us not to fear, not to lose heart. He asks for our complete trust. It may seem at times like we are carrying our cross alone, but He assures us that we need only take our places and stand firm, to trust in Him, and that He will be with us to deliver us. He is doing the fighting for us in the difficulties and challenges of life. Our greatest suffering seems to arise from our submission to our own unfounded fear and anxiety.

We need to ask Jesus to increase and sustain our trust in Him, and then cooperate a bit with the specials graces which He will certainly bestow upon us in response to this prayer. Once we let go of our fears with His help, our suffering is greatly tempered, and we find the joy and peace He wishes to bestow on us. Trusting, though not always easy, is a decision, an act of the will. It is extremely helpful to often pray, "Jesus, I trust in You!" We can only find peace through trusting in God. The greater the degree of trust, the more peace we experience. And our trust will never be in vain. This is certain!

Yes, one may think or say regarding their cancer or adversity that it is more than they can handle. I understand. Even people of great faith can be tempted to think that their cross is too heavy to bear and that God must have made a mistake in their case. True, we may be tested beyond what we think our capacity is, but we will never be tested beyond our true capability. We can count on the wisdom of God here. "The trials you have had to bear are no more than people normally have. You can trust God not to let you be tried beyond your strength, and with any trial he will give you a way out of it and the strength to bear it" (1 Corinthians 10:13, JB). This is a beautiful assurance and consolation that we can take to the bank.

Keep reminding yourself, "Abba, You are with me and You love me. Thank You. You created me. Thank You. You sent Your Son, Jesus, to die for me and save me. Thank You. You sent Your Holy Spirit upon me to shower me with Your gifts! Thank You. I have you, Jesus, so I have everything. Mary, you are my Mother and Queen, constantly presenting my needs to Jesus, which He never refuses to you. Come, Holy Spirit, and own me—use me. Thank You, *Daddy*."

Why Daddy? That is the translation of *Abba*.[19] God wants a profound personal relationship with each of us. His love for each of us is infinite. Perhaps it would be helpful for us in prayer to address our Merciful Father as Daddy or Abba, which I think will make us more aware of our close relationship with Him. A good Daddy is always loving His children and working for their good.

> Paul, an apostle of Christ Jesus by the will of God, and Timothy our brother, to the church of God that is in Corinth, with all the holy ones throughout Achaia: grace to you and peace from God our Father and the Lord Jesus Christ.
>
> Blessed be the God and Father of our Lord Jesus Christ, the Father of compassion and God of all encouragement, who encourages us in our every affliction, so that we may be able to encourage those who are in any affliction with the encouragement with which we ourselves are encouraged by God. For as Christ's sufferings overflow to us, so through Christ does our encouragement also overflow. If we are afflicted, it is for your encouragement and salvation; if we are encouraged, it is for your encouragement, which enables you to endure the same sufferings that we suffer. Our hope for you is firm, for we know that as you share in the sufferings, you also share in the encouragement.
>
> We do not want you to be unaware, brothers, of the affliction that came to us in the province of Asia; we were utterly weighed down beyond our strength, so that we despaired even of life. Indeed, we had accepted within ourselves the sentence of death, that we might trust not in ourselves but in God who raises the dead. He rescued us from such great danger of death, and he will continue to rescue us; in him we have put our hope [that] he will also rescue us again, as you help us with prayer, so that thanks

may be given by many on our behalf for the gift granted us through the prayers of many.

2 Corinthians 1:1–11

Yes, our Father, our Daddy, is the God of compassion and all encouragement. We can't even fathom how much He loves and cares for us. He knows best. Perhaps one of His reasons for permitting our illnesses or other afflictions is so that we may be able to encourage those who are in any affliction with the encouragement with which we ourselves are encouraged by God. Sometimes just a smile, an empathetic touch, or a kind word can mean the world to another beloved child of God.

We are invited to the happy way of trusting in God, not ourselves. We need to ask the Holy Spirit to increase the theological virtue of hope in us. We are called to be positive, and we need to be people of thanksgiving. It is good to focus on the many blessings in our lives each day. It is advantageous to see the cup half-full. When we worry and obsess about our difficulties and troubles we weigh ourselves down in spirit. Most of our suffering derives from our anxiety. We can be less anxious, with God's help, when we make the effort to be positive, to be grateful people, and to look for ways to make others happy, rather than centering on ourselves.

To sum up everything, the answer to every question, doubt, or fear is to trust in Jesus. Though we are incredibly weak and fearful on our own, when we trust Him, with His always present help, we become unshakable. "Those who trust in Yahweh are like Mount Zion, unshakeable, standing forever" (Psalm 125:1, JB). We give Jesus our trust, and He makes a *mountain fortress* out of us; and this fortress is protected by Jesus Himself. "The Hebrew root of the word Zion means landmark, and is often translated as fortress, as according to the Book of Samuel it was the location of the Jebusite fortress conquered by King David."[20]

God, our Loving Father, please help us never to doubt Your care and presence. "Commit your way to the LORD;/ trust that God will act" (Psalm 37:5). With You, Father, we truly have no cause for worries or fears, because You are at all times seeing to our safety, to our healing, seeing to everything for our good. Please grant us the grace to believe and come back to Your Word, Your promise, and to allow You to pick us up when in our human frailty we doubt:

> Hear me, O house of Jacob,/ all who remain of the house of Israel,/ My burden since your birth,/ whom I have carried from your infancy./ Even to your old age I am the same,/ even when your hair is gray I will bear you;/ It is I who have done this, I who will continue,/ and I who will carry you to safety.

> Isaiah 46:3–4

God's love and care for us is eternal. He carries us to safety from infancy to old age, from conception to natural death.

HEALING AS REGARDS FAMILY AND FRIENDS

"Let love be sincere; hate what is evil, hold on to what is good; love one another with mutual affection; anticipate one another in showing honor. Do not grow slack in zeal, be fervent in spirit, serve the Lord. Rejoice in hope, endure in affliction, persevere in prayer. Contribute to the needs of the holy ones, exercise hospitality" (Romans 12:9–13).

Once, my daughter Shealagh, age four at the time, one of the little prophets in our family, came up to me spontaneously and said, "God loves you very much because you bless your children every night." Wow! I have made it my practice for many years to bless each of my children at bedtime with holy water, making a Sign of the Cross on each of their foreheads, saying simply, "God bless you in the name of the Father, and of the Son, and of the Holy Spirit. Amen." When we make a little effort to bring prayer and faith into the family, God rewards us greatly. Our sense of the value of these things is usually heightened when we experience a cross such as cancer.

In July 2010, by the grace of God my family overcame fear, which tends to paralyze and prevent so much good in our lives and the world, as we boldly ventured out on a pilgrimage as a family to visit Niagara Falls in New York, then the Shrine of the North American Martyrs in New York (I was diagnosed with leukemia on their Memorial, October 19, 2009), then the Shrine of Divine Mercy in Massachusetts, and then the St. Joseph Oratory in Montreal, Canada. Our border crossing was interesting as the border police did not initially know what to make of us with such a large number of passengers in our fifteen-seat van purporting to be one large family. After lengthy interviews we won them over and even had them smiling. As we entered Canada, we encountered beautiful rays of the sun emanating through the clouds, welcoming us on our way to St. Joseph's Oratory.

When we had been thinking of going on this pilgrimage, we had initially decided against it due to my poor health and low platelets. But what is life without taking some risks for something worthy? So we spontaneously decided to go late one morning and hastily packed, leaving that same day. Everything went very well. The trip was extraordinarily memorable and grace-filled beyond description. Plus, the kids got to go swimming in a pool every evening at hotels along the way. It was a beautiful family time enriched by our remarkable faith experiences.

We ran out of money before arriving at our last destination, Montreal, but my adult daughter Grace stepped out in faith and loaned us her entire meager life's savings so we could complete the trip. Once we returned home I was able to pay her back within a week with God's always available help.

My illness has also given me much more time to be with my family as I have often been limited in my ability to leave the house. It has had a healing effect on me in that it has heightened my priority of my family first, after God. Though God has not made an angel out of me, I have been able to apply this priority to my life of being with them, trying to be a better husband and father, and being less self-centered. I understand much better the value of spending time with my wife and children. The old adage is true that in retrospect our children grow up fast. I can't emphasize enough that we will never pass this way again.

I have been given the gift of recognizing much more profoundly the precious, unique gems that my wife and each of my children are. I can truly say that when I look, really look, at their faces, I see the Face of God, and this can be overpowering.

Although I fail often, I am motivated to try to be more virtuous, loving, and less of a cross to others, especially my own immediate family members. Of course, my illness sometimes contributes to making me even worse, more tired and irritable, so I remain a cross to them, but I hope I am fighting the good fight (see 1 Timothy 6:12).

The cross is the most effective means God uses to purify us. It is interesting that when I am the sickest I tend to be the most virtuous, being given the grace, through suffering, to see in my neighbors, starting with my own family members, the beautiful image and likeness of God they truly are. My passions are subdued, and the higher faculties of my soul take the lead like they are supposed to. Unfortunately, once I feel stronger and healthier I tend to fall back into my old habits, including impatience, mostly with the ones closest to me, my family members. Lord, help me to love at all times. I am only capable of this tall order with Your help, which I know is never lacking. "If you ask anything of me in my name, I will do it" (John 14:14). I am begging, Lord!

I have also been changed for the better in being motivated to more quickly forgive (though I unfortunately still don't always forgive as immediately as I should) the real or imagined transgression of others against me, knowing that my life could end at any time, and that the opportunity to forgive would be past. God always stands ready to give us the grace to forgive, if we only exercise our free will to ask for His help. Then it is a matter of willing and deciding to forgive, though we may still feel a strong movement of emotions to the contrary. We cannot always control our emotions. We may have to keep exercising our will to forgive many times over, but each time we do, we have in truth forgiven the other person.

I am also motivated by the fact that God will only forgive us if we forgive others, which is only fair. How can we expect mercy if we will not extend it to others? "If you forgive others their transgressions, your heavenly Father will forgive you. But if you do not forgive others, neither will your Father forgive your transgressions" (Matthew 6:14–15). I do not want to die with unforgiveness weighing down my soul. Besides, the one who is most hurt by lack of forgiveness is the one holding the grudge. Lack of forgiveness eats us alive from the inside. It does a great deal of harm to us spiritually as well as psychologically. There is a great healing and peace that comes to the one who forgives.

Another offshoot of my illness is that it has brought the healing of a greater love and relationship from my family members toward me. Their affection has grown, and has often been demonstrated by making sacrificial efforts to help me, and to help with the responsibilities of the household and the younger children. It has made them better and wiser persons. They have grown in their ability to see and to live by what is most important in life. My wife, Kathleen, and I have especially had many profound discussions on this topic. Our love and empathy has grown (if that is possible as it was so great to begin with) for each other and for our children and vice versa.

Another byproduct of my cancer is the numerous friends and family members far and wide, even in other countries, who have been praying and sacrificing for me. I suspect that my illness has been a catalyst for them in many cases to pray more than they otherwise would have, thereby bringing them ever closer to God. Not only that, I suspect that my illness has been a stimulus to confront their own mortality in a more forthright way than they had done before. We should not obsess or be anxious about our mortality, but keeping it in mind certainly helps us to be better persons, and to make the most out of this precious gift of life. I think many were likely helped, by being aware of my situation, to reflect and act upon what were the true priorities in their lives.

This is *all God's work*. "It is you who have accomplished all we have done" (Isaiah 26:12).

I know of one friend in particular who said to our mutual friend something to the effect that he wasn't sure about the existence of God, but that just in case he was praying for me. This is from a man who was apparently not previously the praying type. He is, by the way, an exceptionally virtuous man in many ways.

Edited excerpts from my diary:

> November 4, 2010, St. Charles Borromeo, Bishop: The Ordinary Time Mass reading was the following: "[But] whatever gains I had, these I have come to consider a loss because of Christ. More than that, I even consider everything as a loss because of the supreme good of knowing Christ Jesus my Lord. For his sake I have accepted the loss of all things and I consider them so much rubbish, that I may gain Christ" (Philippians 3:7–8).
>
> This is in line with what I was saying to Kathleen from the depths of my soul a couple weeks ago. I was saying that everything else besides God and family are garbage (rubbish). This is not to be taken literally, but makes the point about what is truly important, and what we should focus our time and energies on.
>
> May we all live each day as if our last and as the gift it is. May we each place God first, and slow down to enable ourselves to see the Face of God in others, especially in our family members. As I walked with my five-year-old, Brighde, the other day, it struck me how she noticed each flower, bird, etc., along the way and would randomly stop to experience these things, while I was initially anxiously trying to move the walk along and get it accomplished. I realized, of course, that she had the right approach. I am very much enjoying how my illness has slowed me down a

bit, and allowed me to wonderfully experience and learn so much more, especially from my own little children.

As parents to our children we are called to simply *be present* to them. Nothing will substitute for our time, presence, and attention devoted to our children.

This is an edited article which I wrote a few years ago for Catholic.net entitled *Fatherhood Moment*:

Scenario: The father of a number of children arrives home from work stressed and exhausted. After greeting his wife, first one child, then the next children in rapid, overpowering succession approach him with a joyful greeting and their need for his attention, their father's irreplaceable attention. One after the other they have something to tell him about their day, perhaps an experience they had at school. For each it is something of great interest. They have a deep need and desire to share with their father.

A grand occasion has been presented by God our Father's good providence. This dad has been given an opportunity to emulate Him in virtues such as magnanimity, patience, selfless listening, and in giving. Our Father in heaven is a *giver* by his very nature. He is a *pourer*, while we can naturally tend to be *drippers*, or shall we say *drips*. A *pourer* is one who gives everything, all that he is, and all that he has to God and others, swiftly, without holding back.

First case in point: Dad is basically a good man with good intentions, but he takes no time to pray or to plan how he will live those first moments when he arrives home. When his children approach him he cuts them off, "Not now, I'm busy!" The wind leaves their sails. Perhaps the children do not let on that they are disappointed, but the damage is done. The wound has been struck. His children had something important to share with their one and only daddy because of their singular love and respect for him. Yet the opportunity is missed. Though there will be others, this God-given opportunity is lost. This providential occasion will never exactly repeat itself. What just happened is locked in time. In this case Dad made the grim error of thinking and acting as if there was something more important than providing his full attention to each child for a few moments.

Second case in point: Dad is well aware of his weakness and tendencies. So he has prepared. He took five minutes to pray just before arriving home, shoring himself up with desperately needed graces. He also took time to visualize these most important first ten minutes with his family when he arrives home. He has a plan of what he will do and how he will act. He has made a resolution to serve and to *pour* himself out, rather than to act like the self-centered *drip* he knows he can so easily be—instead of expecting to be served. He is barraged with multiple children, perhaps one at a time, perhaps more than one at a time, starving for and demanding his attention. It is a little overwhelming, as he struggles with his selfishness, stress, and tiredness, but he says a quick prayer for divine assistance, and valiantly, manfully holds fast to his resolution and plan.

One of his daughters in particular has a story to tell from school that seems to go on and on with more details than he could ever imagine. The story confuses him, and tests his stamina. Yet, through an act of the will, with divine assistance, he gives his complete, cheerful attention, without interruption, with eyes and ears riveted on this child and on each child in turn, until they have had their full opportunity to express themselves. Then one of his daughters, the one that told the longest story, the one who really tested his resolve, gives him a hug and says, "Daddy, you're the best daddy in the world!" Though he knows this is not true, he thanks his Father of Mercies for giving him the grace to at least live these few moments well. After all, isn't this the stuff of life, seemingly little moments, but in actuality big opportunities to live love, or to choose not do so? It comes down to a question of being a *pourer* or being a *drip*. With prayer and a little planning, effort, courage, and tenacity we can be the pourers, the other Christs our Father wants us to be.

"Yahweh, you are our Father; we the clay, you the potter, we are all the work of your hand" (Isaiah 64:7–8, JB). *Father*, what a profound word!

Our Father—this is how Christ taught us to address our infinite God. We are called and offered the graces to emulate our Father in heaven. "The divine fatherhood is the source of human fatherhood"[21] (CCC 2214).

Flash ahead forty years. How quickly they have passed! This father's body lies in his casket at the funeral home surrounded by his family. His time is up. His life has been poured out. His children pour out their love and praises of their father to each person coming to pay their respects. They all go on repeating to everyone that their father was the best father anyone could ever hope for. He always made time to be present and to listen to his children at any cost to himself. "Well done, good and faithful servant."

Matthew 25:23, JB

The father of a family is indispensable. He leads and serves. He is the head of the family, but in the sense that he is the head to the degree that he serves and sacrifices. He is the living, active image of Christ on the cross to his wife and children. "Husbands should love their wives just as Christ loved the Church and sacrificed himself for her to make her holy" (Ephesians 5:25–26, JB).

The Church proclaims the profound truth that marriage is indissoluble. Like Jesus, whose bride is the Church, we are called to stay with our spouse until death. This commitment becomes attainable with the graces that are always available from the Sacrament of Matrimony. If God asks something of us, He always gives us the help we need to complete our mission. We need more finishers is the world. Jesus did not desert His mission when the going got tough. He expected it and embraced it. Marriage can be challenging in many ways. What would we think of a soldier who enjoyed the benefits of being in the military during peacetime, but who deserted at the first sign of battle?

> The love of the spouses requires, of its very nature, the unity and indissolubility of the spouses' community of persons, which embraces their entire life: "so they are no longer two, but one flesh."[22] They "are called to grow continually in their communion through day-to-day fidelity to their marriage promise of total mutual self-giving."
>
> CCC 1644[23]

I think that cancer and other serious adversities give us a greater appreciation for our spouse. We often experience the self-giving of our spouse as our caregiver. We experience how when one suffers, so does the other out of a deep empathy, deeper than any human bond, because we have truly become one.

And a special word for men, since I am one of you. Our wives and children need us, faults and all. We are irreplaceable. Let's be the noble knights God wants us to be and stick with our wives no matter what, and that means no exceptions. God made us inherently warriors of a sort. Just watch young boys playing, how they will quite naturally turn sticks into pretend guns or swords. We should channel the fight that is in us to love, sacrifice for, and protect our wives through thick and thin. It is God to whom we made a *vow* when we became united in matrimony with our wives. "So then, what God has united, man must not divide" (Mark 10:9–10, jb).

Children need their fathers on numerous levels. For one, he has the God-appointed mission of being the spiritual and moral leader of his family.

> Happy are all who fear the Lord,/ who walk in the ways of God./ What your hands provide you will enjoy;/ you will be happy and prosper:/ Like a fruitful vine/ your wife within your home,/ Like olive plants/ your children around your table./ Just so will they be blessed/ who fear the Lord.
>
> Psalm 128:1–4

There are many sacrifices a good father offers for his family, such as working hard to provide for them, giving of his time to be with them, doing yard work, you name it. There is something more that must be done, however. He can offer all of his sacrifices—and in the case of having cancer he can offer that up to God—through prayer to be made one with the sacrifice, suffering, and death of Jesus for the spiritual and corporal good of his family. This is a noble thing.

Wives are called to be the heart of their families and to never give up. When a heart stops beating the body dies. When the wife/mom is not present, loving, and serving the family, the body of the family becomes decimated.

None of us is expected to be perfect on a human level. What counts in the end is the effort and commitment that is persevered in.

When we encounter a severe cross, we are healed so as to be able to comprehend the things that are most important in our lives, such as our children. *What are the four greatest gifts parents can give to their children?* Sure, as parents we are called to do our best in providing for our children including housing, food, clothing, and education. How about making star athletes out of our children at the cost of our family always being harried, busy, rushed, and exhausted, having little down time to enjoy family unity and peace? Are these among the supreme gifts? No! I maintain that the *first of the greatest gifts* is to pass on the gift of faith in God, leading by example, including the unswerving practice of one's faith and religion.

The *second greatest gift* is a secure, enduring, happy marriage between father and mother. The children find a great sense of security in this, and they will flourish more in virtually every aspect of their lives. This calls for commitment, effort, and sacrificial love on the part of the parents.

The *third greatest gift* is something children ask for often. When the gift is received the entire family is incredibly joyful and transformed on the special occasion of this magnificent gift. The family will never be the same. The gift calls for courage and generosity on the part of the givers. The gift lasts for many decades, only getting better, changing, and developing each day. The gift is unique, and can never be repeated, but a similar gift can be added approximately every year. It can only be given by three persons agreeing and acting. Yes, the profound gift is that of another child. And those three persons are husband, wife, and God.

The *fourth greatest gift* is that of the parents, to the best of their ability, and at the cost of sacrificing many things, being *present* to and loving their children. No amount of money, gifts, sports, or activities will ever be able to substitute for our loving presence with our children.

September 24, 2011: This morning while I was praying in my bedroom, my daughter Brighde, age six, came in as she often does and lay on her back on the carpeted floor. It was a precious gem of a moment. She said, "I love laying on your floor," as she made herself extremely comfortable. It was to me as if she had said, "I love the security and love I feel being in your presence, Daddy."

Thank You, Jesus, for the gift of my family and friends and these particular gifts of grace. Oh, how they lift me up to You!

May I conclude this chapter with a prayer I composed that I wish to recommend for married couples to pray together frequently:

Dear Most Holy Trinity, Father, Son, and Holy Spirit, thank You for the profound gift of the Sacrament of Marriage. Thank You for the magnificent gift of my spouse whom Your perfect providence planned for me from all eternity. May I always treat him (her) as royalty, with all the perfect honor, respect, and dignity he (she) deserves. Help me to be selfless in my marriage, to pour everything out for my spouse at all times, holding nothing back, expecting nothing in return, but recognizing and being grateful for all he (she) pours out for me and our family every day, and it is much! Please strengthen and protect our marriage and all marriages. Help us to pray together daily. May we trust You completely in every way, as You deserve. Please make our marriage fruitful and open to Your most perfect will in the privilege of cocreating and nurturing life. Help us to build a strong, secure, loving, faith-filled family, the domestic church. Dear Most Blessed Virgin Mary, we confidently entrust our marriage to your care. Keep our family always under your mantle. We have complete trust in You, Lord Jesus, that You are always with us, and are constantly seeing to the very best for us, bringing a tremendous good out of everything, including the crosses you have permitted in our lives. Dear (spouse's name): You and I are one. I promise I will always love you, and always be true to you. I will never abandon you. I will lay down my life for you. With God and you in my life I have everything. Thank You, Jesus. You are the ultimate "Pourer." We love you.

HEALING
AS REGARDS OTHERS

"Blessed be the God and Father of our Lord Jesus Christ, the Father of compassion and God of all encouragement, who encourages us in our every affliction, so that we may be able to encourage those who are in any affliction with the encouragement with which we ourselves are encouraged by God. For as Christ's sufferings overflow to us, so through Christ does our encouragement also overflow" (2 Corinthians 1:3–5).

"No foul language should come out of your mouths, but only such as is good for needed edification, that it may impart grace to those who hear. And do not grieve the holy Spirit of God, with which you were sealed for the day of redemption. All bitterness, fury, anger, shouting, and reviling must be removed from you, along with all malice. be kind to one another, compassionate, forgiving one another as God has forgiven you in Christ" (Ephesians 4:29–32).

> Edited excerpts from my diary: June 15, 2009: Last night I dreamt of driving my car in Chicago, and that somehow I dropped an unopened bottle of beer on the floor, and I couldn't reach it. It had rolled under the passenger seat. In the morning I heard on the radio (and also read later in the newspaper) that a woman from the South Side

of Chicago was charged with DUI after crashing into a viaduct on Saturday, while allegedly reaching for a bottle of "alcohol," and that her nine-year-old daughter's head hit the windshield. There, but for the grace of God, go I. When I have an occasional dream like this I deduce that God wants me to pray for the people involved, which I did.

October 18, 2009: The First Reading at Mass is Isaiah 53:10–11: "[But the LORD was pleased/ to crush him in infirmity.]/ If he gives his life as an offering for sin,/ he shall see his descendants in a long life,/ and the will of the LORD shall be accomplished through him./ Because of his affliction/ he shall see the light in fullness of days;/ Through his suffering, my servant shall justify many,/ and their guilt he shall bear."

Also, the gospel at Mass today was Mark 10:38: "Can you drink the cup that I drink…?" I had long ago told Jesus, "Yes, I can drink the cup; Your will be done."

October 19, 2009: Memorial of SS. Isaac Jogues and John de Brébeuf, priests and martyrs, and Companions, martyrs. I received a provisional diagnosis of Chronic Lymphocytic Leukemia. Not my will, but Yours be done.

This is also the one-year anniversary of Louis and Zelie Martin (parents of St. Thérèse of Lisieux) being proclaimed Blessed (the last step before canonization) by the Catholic Church. Kathleen and I have many parallels with them, though they were ideal examples, parallels we have tried to live in our family, often falling very short. God is so good and merciful.

The Office of Readings quotes St. John de Brébeuf: "I will take from your hand the cup of your sufferings and call upon your name."[24] I had long ago given myself to Jesus in the Mass offering to *drink of the cup* according to His will. Not that I necessarily asked for suffering or death, but only to fulfill His will to make myself totally available to Him in freedom, whether in suffering, death, or a long life of trying to serve Him and souls.

Jesus is more than with us. He is in us, and we are in Him. He experiences deeply, empathetically, and in actuality everything we experience. We are one with Him, and He is one with us. Jesus has consecrated Himself for us. "And I consecrate myself for them, so that they also may be consecrated in truth. I pray not only for them, but also for those who will believe in me through their word, so that they may all be one, as you, Father, are in me and I in you, that they also may be in us, that the world may believe that you sent me" (John 17:19–21). Whatever happens to the least of us happens to Jesus Himself. "Amen, I say to you, whatever you did for one of these least brothers of mine, you did for me" (Matthew 25:40). Whenever any one of us suffers, Jesus is really, and in a mystical way, suffering in His oneness in us, since each of us is, at least implicitly, a member of His Mystical Body.[25]

In Acts 9:2 we see Saul (who is later known as Paul) persecuting the Church, "that, if he should find any men or women who belonged to the Way, he might bring them back to Jerusalem in chains." Here was Saul who was involved in the stoning of the first martyr, Deacon Stephen, and who was trying to destroy the Church.

> Now Saul was consenting to his [Stephen's] execution. On that day, there broke out a severe persecution of the church in Jerusalem, and all were scattered throughout the countryside of Judea and Samaria, except the apostles.... Saul, meanwhile, was trying to destroy the church; entering house after house dragging out men and women, he handed them over for imprisonment.
>
> Acts 8:1, 3

In Acts, chapter 9, we see Saul knocked off his horse, so to speak, by the Lord Jesus. Jesus said, "'Saul, why are you persecuting me?' He said, 'Who are you, sir?' The reply came, 'I am Jesus, whom you are persecuting'" (Acts 9:4–5). I borrow an insight from Venerable Archbishop Fulton J. Sheen, which I often do. How could Saul be persecuting Jesus if Jesus had died, risen, ascended into heaven, and is seated at the right hand of the Father?[26] By the way, we see in Acts 7:56 that Jesus always stands to defend whenever a member of His Mystical Body is persecuted or suffers:[27] "Behold, I see the heavens opened and the Son of Man standing at the right hand of God" (Acts 7:56). He is one with us.

So we see that Jesus identifies with each of us as one with us in our suffering. When we suffer so does Jesus suffer in His Mystical Body, and this suffering is not a waste! It is purifying and redemptive! It is power!

Venerable Archbishop Fulton J. Sheen used to visit a sick person and ask for a few minutes of his or her prayers before he preached.[28] Some of the power and grace of the prayers and suffering of the sick person were transferred to Archbishop Sheen. He acknowledged that all of his power came from Jesus in the Eucharist and from the suffering persons who interceded for him. And he was truly filled with the power of the Holy Spirit!

Dear reader, Jesus loves you infinitely and is with you every step of the way. I am sure He is proud of your fortitude and endurance in this battle, which is only for the good including your own purification and to contribute to the work of redemption for many others, first and foremost your own family members. "Now I rejoice in my sufferings for your sake, and in my flesh I am filling up what is lacking in the afflictions of Christ on behalf of his body, which is the church" (Colossians 1:24–25).

Yes, the merits of our sufferings and prayers are transferable to others, those living on earth, and those completing their purification in purgatory before entering the eternal heavenly banquet. To borrow and expound upon an idea from Venerable

Archbishop Fulton Sheen, if it is possible to transfuse blood from one person to another to save that person's life, it is most certainly possible in the spiritual realm for God to permit the transference of the merits of prayer and suffering from one to another in His Mystical Body.[29]

I find it interesting that one who donates blood will usually never know the identity of the recipient of the charitable act. Those of us who offer our prayers and sufferings for others will often not know the identity of all of the recipients of these graces. Sometimes the person receiving the blood transfusion is unconscious and helpless. Just so, many recipients of these transferable graces are unable to help themselves. It takes the faith, prayer, and sufferings or sacrifices of another to lift that soul up to God for redemption and healing. We are our brother's keeper.

We can be absolutely certain that when we pray selflessly for the true good of another person, that prayer will always be answered in the affirmative, though God is the final determiner of whether what we think of as good is truly good for that person, with an eye on his or her eternal salvation. What we think is good may not be so good. In that case God will give something even better instead. Prayer is powerful and never wasted.

The power of prayer comes from God and returns back to Him when we pray, only to be replenished in us in an even greater proportion. Prayer always gets results, always! I am convinced that when we pray and sacrifice fervently for the spiritual good of another, such as his or her salvation or conversion, we can have no doubt that the intention for which we are praying will be granted. It is then not a question of *if* the prayer petition will be granted for the good of this other soul, but *when* God sees as the best time.

God's time is typically not our time. He is patient, and so should we be. We should have absolute faith and confidence in the efficacy of our prayers and sacrifices, and in God's goodness. I like to end my prayers with "The mountain has been cast into the sea!" from the following Bible passage: "Jesus answered, 'Have faith in

God. I tell you solemnly, if anyone says to this mountain, "Get up and throw yourself into the sea," with no hesitation in his heart but believing that what he says will happen, it will be done for him. I tell you therefore: everything you ask and pray for, believe that you have it already, and it will be yours…'" (Mark 11:23–25, JB). Note that it is God who responds to the prayer and gets the results for us. What magnificent power He has gifted us with in prayer! May we never neglect or waste this power, for the good of ourselves and others.

When we pray we should trust that God is good and faithful. Any other attitude would be to wound His Sacred Heart, which always overflows with love and goodness. How could He not grant the good of another soul when we pray? This would be against His very nature, and therefore impossible.

When God permits a serious cross such as cancer in our lives it is truly a stupendous gift for our good and the good of others, resulting in His glory. I do not want to be disingenuous and claim that the cross is all rosy and wonderful, or that those of us who are hanging and bleeding there should be outwardly happy and asserting how wonderful it is. No. The cross is the cross. It is hard. It was hard for Him to hang there and bleed.[30] And it is hard for us to hang there when Christ lifts us up *to hang there with Him*. But deep down in the superior part of our soul there is to be found a spiritual joy.

The cross would have no value separated from the resurrection. The resurrection and our very salvation is the fruit of the tree of the cross. And believe me when I tell you that your cross is bearing fruit in your salvation and that of others. Jesus has privileged us with a tiny share of His cross with which to contribute to His mission of saving mankind. We will be eternally grateful for our crosses.

Our Blessed Lord Jesus Himself did not have to suffer and die for us. "This is why the Father loves me, because I lay down my life in order to take it up again. No one takes it from me, but I lay it down on my own. I have power to lay it down, and power to take it up again. This command I have received from my Father" (John 10:17–18). Imagine that—choosing to suffer in this way when He could have saved Himself at any time. How many of us would choose to suffer if we could avoid it? His is not human love, but divine. And Jesus has *divinized us* through His death and resurrection and by sending His Holy Spirit to reside in us.

Yes, we are actually incorporated and transformed into Christ, and thereby divinized, so that the Father sees Jesus when He looks at us. We become the *smell of a fertile field*, a fragrant aroma to Him. "He blessed him saying: 'Yes, the smell of my son is like the smell of a fertile field blessed by Yahweh'" (Genesis 27:27, JB). This divinization "is all God's work" (2 Corinthians 5:17–18, JB).

We are each made into another Christ, not equal to Jesus of course, but another Jesus nonetheless.

> The Word became flesh to make us *"partakers of the divine nature."*[31] "For this is why the Word became man, and the Son of God became the Son of man: so that man, by entering into communion with the Word and thus receiving divine sonship, might become a son of God."[32] "For the Son of God became man so that we might become God."[33] "The only-begotten Son of God, wanting to make us sharers in his divinity, assumed our nature, so that he, made man, might make men gods."[34]
>
> CCC 460

Edited excerpt from my diary: March 9, 2008: It may have been in a dream last night. Someone said that I need to be a Cyrenean (to help Christ and others carry their crosses). In my meditation in the morning the next passage in my Bible was Matthew 27:32–33 (JB) about Simon the Cyrenean.

"On their way out, they came across a man from Cyrene,
Simon by name, and enlisted him to carry his cross."

It is interesting that the "chief local export (of Cyrene) through
much of its early history was the medicinal herb silphium, used
to induce an abortion (referred in the medical community to
as an abortifacient); the herb was pictured on most Cyrenian
coins."[35] Perhaps there is a secondary apropos message in this
Gospel passage wherein there was a need for reparation by a
Cyrenean, a Christ figure, for the sin of the myriad of abortions
the Cyreneans were complicit with. Scripture contains an infinite
number of treasures to be hunted and discovered with the help of
the Holy Spirit.

We are called to be Cyreneans, to help Jesus to carry His cross
by carrying ours, to contribute to our own salvation and that of all
mankind. This is our Loving Father's perfect will. "This command
I have received from my Father" (John 10:18).

And when they had mocked him, they stripped him of the
purple cloak, dressed him in his own clothes, and led him
out to crucify him. They pressed into service a passer-by,
Simon, a Cyrenian, who was coming in from the country,
the father of Alexander and Rufus, to carry his cross.

Mark 15:20–21

In a practical sense we can facilitate healing for others by
offering those we encounter a smile, a kind deed, a kind word, by
asking them sincerely how things are going in their lives, really
listening empathetically, and offering our presence and words of
encouragement. This will mean much to others, especially when
they know it is coming from someone who is bearing a heavy cross
of their own. The gospels are full of examples of the empathy of
Jesus, which we are called to emulate.

A leper came to him [and kneeling down] begged him and said, "If you wish, you can make me clean." Moved with pity, he stretched out his hand, touched him, and said to him, "I do will it. Be made clean." The leprosy left him immediately, and he was made clean.

Mark 1:40–42

It is hard to fathom, but Jesus was concerned with others even while He hung on the cross, such as when He forgave those who crucified Him. And He desires that we emulate Him in this manner. "Father, forgive them, they know not what they do" (Luke 23:34). And He empathizes with, encourages, and awards the good thief who was being crucified at His side. "Then he said, 'Jesus, remember me when you come into your kingdom' He replied to him, 'Amen, I say to you, today you will be with me in Paradise'" Luke 23:42–43).

Through my cancer I have been presented with many opportunities to help others that never would have presented themselves in my normal routine of life before my illness. In particular I have met numerous wonderful people at Northwestern Memorial Hospital where I received almost all of my treatment. God has healed me in the sense of my being able to step out of my bubble and engage and be concerned about others around me, which would not normally be my nature.

For example, I now try to engage those around me with an authentic smile or friendly word much more often than I did before. The Lord Jesus inspired me to pass out Divine Mercy holy cards, to as many people as possible that I encounter, for instance, clerks at stores who serve me. I would estimate that approximately 95 percent have accepted the cards when I offered them. Some persons appear awestruck and pleasantly overwhelmed by the gift of the holy card. This little gift seems like such a small thing in a sense, but in actual fact it can be, and I believe often is, a truly efficacious spiritual experience in the life of the person receiving it. There are most certainly many graces available for the one receiving when one chooses to accept them.

There are evil spirits at work that labor, often very effectively, to confuse us and instigate fear in us so that we might be persuaded that we should never discuss God or our faith with another, that this might be offensive to the other party, certainly politically incorrect, and that the other person might become angry. The truth is that there is no reason to be afraid. All we are doing is sharing, not imposing, a great gift. This is an act of love. We should never be dissuaded from acts of charity like this.

I am troubled to experience that even after engaging countless others about faith and God to greater and lesser extents over the past two decades, I sometimes still become irrationally timid and hesitant to engage another person about spiritual things. It is very rare that I encounter an angry reaction from someone; and I don't remember a single negative reaction in regard to the Divine Mercy holy card. There is a spiritual battle raging, but we merely need to call on the help of Jesus, to trust in Him, and all will be well.

This Divine Mercy holy card depicts a beautiful image of Jesus. (See the image in Photo Section.)

> In 1931, Our Lord appeared to St. Faustina. She saw Jesus clothed in a white garment with His right hand raised in blessing. His left hand was touching His garment in the area of the heart, from where two large rays came forth, one red and the other pale. She gazed intently at the Lord in silence, her soul filled with awe, but also with great joy. Jesus said to her, "Paint an image according to the pattern you see, with the signature: Jesus, I trust in You…I promise that the soul that will venerate this image will not perish. I also promise victory over [its] enemies already here on earth, especially at the hour of death. I Myself will defend it as My own glory" (Diary 47, 48). "I am offering people

a vessel with which they are to keep coming for graces to the fountain of mercy. That vessel is this image with the signature: 'Jesus, I trust in You.'"

Diary 327[36]

So, by the grace of God, I have been handing these holy cards out to almost every staff member as well as many patients at the hospital, and there have been probably many hundreds of such encounters. I have begun passing out my third box of 500. Numerous hospital staff members have this card posted on a wall or such at their desks.

I have had many opportunities to speak with others about God. Sometimes when I offer a holy card to someone, it results in a conversation about the Lord that never would have otherwise occurred. Another example is that once while I was waiting for treatment at the hospital, one of the receptionists approached me to ask if I would meet with a cancer patient in the chemotherapy section. She explained that this woman was interested in the Divine Mercy devotion, and wanted to see me. She had somehow apparently heard that I pass out Divine Mercy cards. I visited her in a room where she was receiving chemotherapy by IV. I learned from her that she had terminal cancer. She was apparently taking chemo to extend her life. We ended up having a very lengthy and profound talk about faith and God. It turned out that she was Catholic. Through no merit of mine, with the Holy Spirit acting through me, I was able to help and console her. At the end of the visit she asked if I was a hospital chaplain. I told her that I was not, but merely a fellow cancer patient. I thank God for this opportunity to have helped this wonderful, courageous woman, and to be inspired by her. I think this is a case in point wherein if we make ourselves available to God He will use us for the good of others and His glory. Praised be Jesus!

HEALING THROUGH ACCEPTING GOD'S WAYS

"For my thoughts are not your thoughts,/ nor are your ways my ways, says the LORD./ As high as the heavens are above the earth,/ so high are my ways above your ways/ and my thoughts above your thoughts" (Isaiah 55:8–9).

> Edited excerpt from my diary: October 25, 2010, St. Anthony Mary Claret: I can truly say that I love my leukemia. It has been a special healing grace to bring me down into a broken state so that God can lift me up to union with Him. "God, you have rejected us, broken us" (Psalm 60:1, JB).
>
> I also had a sense in my prayer today of the undeniable fact that nothing can touch me, hurt me, or kill me unless and until, as was the case with Himself, Jesus says so.[37] "This is why the Father loves me, because I lay down my life in order to take it up again. No one takes it from me, but I lay it down on my own. I have power to lay it down, and power to take it up again. This command I have received from my Father" (John 10:17–18). Everything is subject to

His perfect will and providence. He is seeing to the perfect
good and timing for each of us. Thank You, Jesus.

We can live in peace when we come to accept God's will in the
many facets of our lives. There is a great freedom and rest in this
surrender! "Come to me, all you who labor and are burdened, and
I will give you rest. Take my yoke upon you and learn from me,
for I am meek and humble of heart; and you will find rest for
yourselves. For my yoke is easy, and my burden light" (Matthew
11:28–30).

Yes, we can never fully understand God because He is God,
and we are not. But, if I may be so bold, I think He does permit us
a generalization which can often be true: God's ways are usually
180 degrees opposite of our ways.

As a practical example, my wife, Kathleen, has been blessed
with nineteen children in eighteen pregnancies. (Quick, how is
that possible? We had one set of twins.) Kathleen was pregnant
with number nineteen when our eldest, Shannon, was nineteen
years old. We were blessed in our marriage with an average of
one child per year. Our ways, the ways of the culture, and the
view of the world would say that she would be a physical, mental,
and emotional wreck. Though I admit there have been many
challenges in bearing and raising so many children, and, yes, I will
admit that our lives are sometimes very crazy and hectic, the joy
and blessings of having a large family have immensely outweighed
the difficulties.

Kathleen is a beautiful, attractive, vibrant woman (she looks at
least ten years younger than her actual age, even being mistaken
at times as a sister to our children as opposed to their mother),
healthy in mind, body, emotions, and spirit. She is a highly
accomplished and loving wife and mother; spiritually blessed
as a daily Mass attendee and woman of prayer and the interior
life; educationally gifted wherein she has a teaching degree, a law
degree, and is currently in the process of pursuing her master's in

theology; professionally accomplished as a Director of Religious Education responsible for over 1200 students; spiritually gifted and generous as a spiritual guide to other women; a talented author with a published book and various articles; a public speaker to thousands on faith and family; as well as a guest numerous times on radio and television.

I could go on, but the reader might become exhausted by my boasting about my wife. God's ways are not our ways. The more we step out in faith and trust in the Most High God, the more we are blessed. The more we give, the more we receive. "Give and gifts will be given to you; a good measure, packed together, shaken down, and overflowing, will be poured into your lap. For the measure with which you measure will in return be measured out to you" (Luke 6:38).

The spirit of the world, personified by the tyrannical definer of political correctness, the anonymous *they* (as in *they say*), would have us believe that children from such a large family as ours could not possibly receive enough love, education, and attention to thrive. Thanks be to God, though far from perfect, all of our children are virtuous and mature well beyond their age. They all have excelled in school, and all of our older children of age have graduated from or are attending private college, all with some level of financial scholarships. Four out of five of our university graduates thus far are pursing or have achieved advanced degrees or certification. All of our children have emerged as leaders; and none have become casualties of the culture. Though they, as do all of us, have their faults, they are living lives of faith, virtue, and chastity. God's ways are not our ways.

How can we begin to understand and accept God's ways? We must seek His Spirit. "Now the natural person does not accept what pertains to the Spirit of God, for to him it is foolishness, and he cannot understand it, because it is judged spiritually. The spiritual person, however, can judge everything but is not subject to judgment by anyone" (1 Corinthians 2:14–15).

Who is the Holy Spirit? He is God, the third Person of the Most Holy Trinity. He unveils Jesus to us.

> "No one comprehends the thoughts of God except the Spirit of God."[38] Now God's Spirit, who reveals God, makes known to us Christ, his Word, his living Utterance, but the Spirit does not speak of himself. The Spirit who "has spoken through the prophets" makes us hear the Father's Word, but we do not hear the Spirit himself. We know him only in the movement by which he reveals the Word to us and disposes us to welcome him in faith. The Spirit of truth who "unveils" Christ to us "will not speak on his own."[39] Such properly divine self-effacement explains why "the world cannot receive [him], because it neither sees him nor knows him," while those who believe in Christ know the Spirit because he dwells with them.[40]

CCC 687

We who have and live the Catholic faith are wholly one in the Holy Spirit. We could say that the Holy Spirit is the Love between the Father and Son personified. He is the Spirit of the Mystical Body of Christ, which consists of the members of His Church. After having been baptized, and more fully when we are confirmed, we receive the Holy Spirit, and are empowered to better understand and live the things of God. We are one with the other members of the Church and with God. You might say we begin to think and act alike, while at the same time retaining our uniqueness.

A very dim reflection of this action of the Spirit is as follows. When I was young I was a rock-and-roll fan. I would occasionally attend concerts. There were other attendees with diverse races and backgrounds, old and young, rich and poor, educated and uneducated. But when the band played we were one in spirit.

This was palpable. This spirit, one might say, was like a burning light. We would all spontaneously light lighters or matches to symbolize this spirit we were experiencing. There was an amazing joy and unity among us. Of course, this experience was ephemeral. Well, if fans at a rock concert can be one in spirit, then certainly God can make us one in His Spirit! This Holy Spirit is lasting and infinitely more effective and transforming. He lights up the Truth, Jesus, for us. He unveils Christ to us. He causes our hearts to burn. "Did not our hearts burn within us...?" (Luke 24:32, JB). He is our All.

When we receive the Holy Spirit we become God's sacred temple where He abides. "The temple of God is sacred; and you are that temple" (1 Corinthians 3:17, JB). This also means that others are temples of the Holy Spirit, and should be treated by us accordingly. They are other Christs. "I tell you solemnly, in so far as you did this to one of these least of these brothers of mine, you did it to me" (Matthew 25:40, JB).

We are members of the Mystical Body of Christ, whose spirit is the Holy Spirit, who unifies His members. "Incorporated into Christ by Baptism, the person baptized is configured to Christ. Baptism seals the Christian with the indelible spiritual mark (character) of his belonging to Christ. No sin can erase this mark, even if sin prevents Baptism from bearing the fruits of salvation."[41] (CCC 1272)

There is another spirit, a divisive spirit, who some choose to follow; though there is always prevailing hope for them. They depend on our help and prayers. Be on guard, but never fear. "Be calm, but vigilant..." (1 Peter 5:8, JB). The devil loses in the end; his days are numbered. "The devil has gone down to you in a rage, knowing that his days are numbered" (Revelation 12:12, JB).

"And I shall put my spirit in you, and you will live, and I shall resettle you on your own soil; and you will know that I, Yahweh, have said and done this—it is the Lord Yahweh who speaks"

(Ezekiel 37:14, JB). It is through the Spirit that we have life. It is God who gifts us with His Spirit. It is through the Spirit that we know that God is the One Who does everything for us. Without Him we are nothing; we can do nothing. "Whoever remains in me, with me in him, bears fruit in plenty; for cut off from me you can do nothing" (John 15:5, JB). It is only through God that we can accomplish our mission of producing fruit with our lives. We do not want to conclude our lives with empty hands, because we want to please our beloved Lord, because we love Him, thanks to the help of His Spirit.

How do we receive the Holy Spirit? We receive Him most importantly through the Sacraments of Baptism and Confirmation and the other Sacraments of the Catholic Church, by which we receive sanctifying grace, but we also receive Him through our prayer. We are then raised above our natural selves and capabilities. We seek His Spirit to be one with our spirit, wherein we can begin to understand and accept God's ways. We receive at least some dim understanding of the things of God, and the grace to believe that all God permits is working toward our good, even though we do not have a complete understanding (because God is God and we are not). It is interesting that God has shared such potent power with us in the gift of free will, that it is the only power that we can say, in a sense, can thwart God's plan, should we exercise it to choose to turn from Him.

The ways of God, His ways, are not our ways. Since He is a loving Father, He will permit challenges in our lives so that we can grow and be healed in untold ways, in the best and most crucial ways.

> You have also forgotten the exhortation addressed to you as sons:/ "My son, do not disdain the discipline of the Lord/ or lose heart when reproved by him;/ for whom the Lord loves, he disciplines;/ he scourges every son he acknowledges." / Endure your trials as "discipline"; God

treats you as sons. For what "son" is there whom his father does not discipline?

Hebrews 12:5–7

To sum it up, God's will *is*. Yes, God's will is what it is. There is nothing that is not enfolded in His providence. I can't proclaim it enough! God's will is perfect, and is bringing a tremendous good out of everything in our lives. "We know that by turning everything to their good, God co-operates with all those who love him" (Romans 8:28, JB).

God's ways are not our ways. His plan will always have a large degree of mystery in it, but we can surely trust that His plan is for the best every time. "Oh, the depth of the riches and wisdom and knowledge of God! How inscrutable are his judgments and how unsearchable his ways! For who has known the mind of the Lord/ or who has been his counselor?" (Romans 11:33–34). Jesus, I trust in You!

PHOTOS

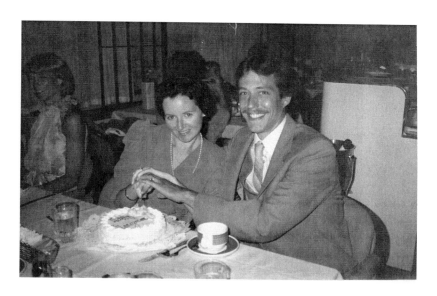

Jim and Kathleen on honeymoon

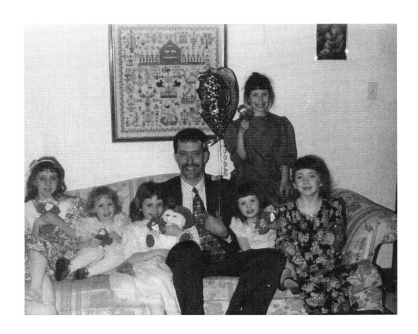

After Daddy Daughter Dance

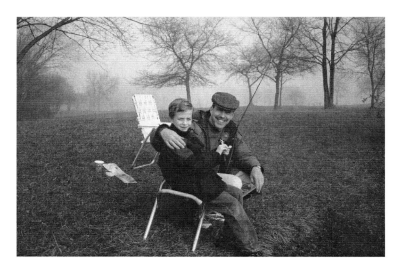

Dad and son, Shane going fishing

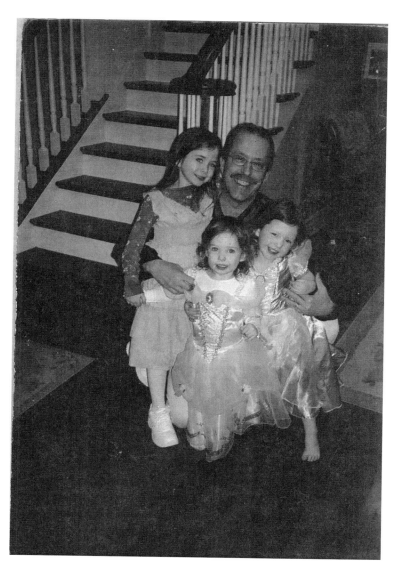

Dad with princesses

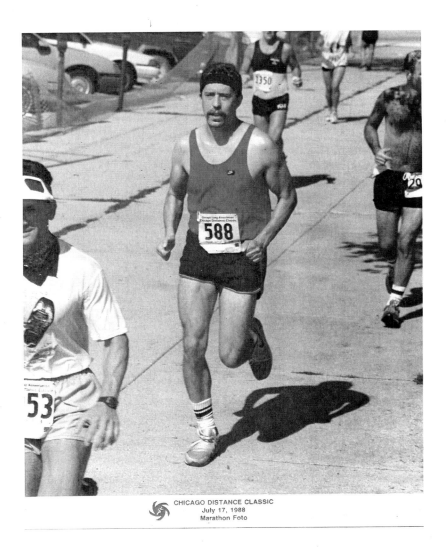

CHICAGO DISTANCE CLASSIC
July 17, 1988
Marathon Foto

He gives strength to the fainting; for the weak
he makes vigor abound Isaiah 40 29

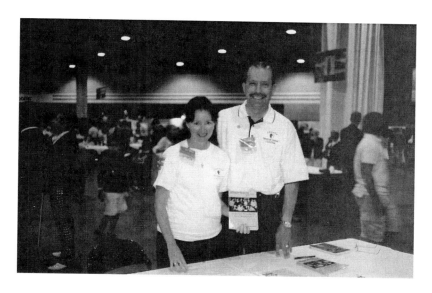

Jim and Kathleen at book signing for Better by the Dozen, Plus Two

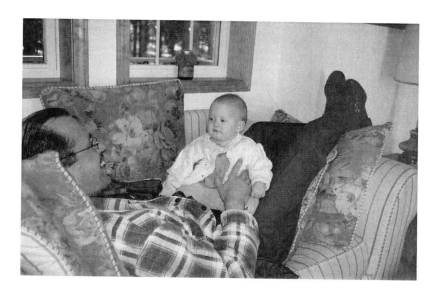

I don't know if I trust this guy

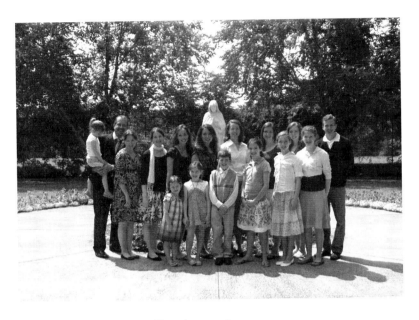

Family togetherness

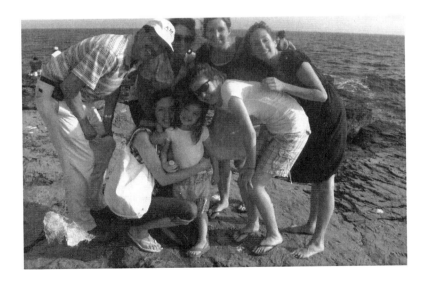

Fun at the ocean

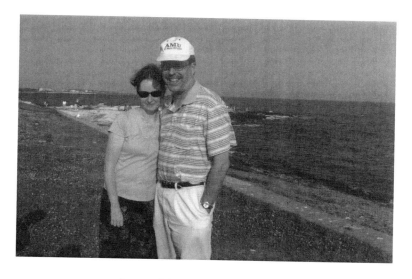

Jim and Kathleen at the ocean

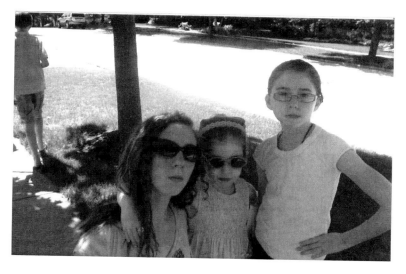

Don't mess with the Littletons

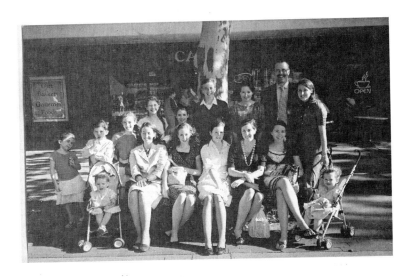

Littletons visiting in Newport, RI

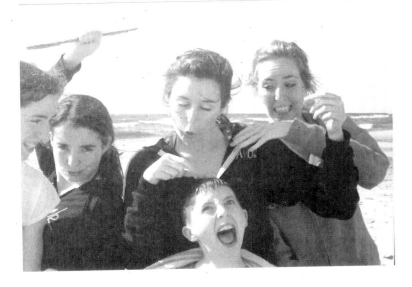

A little crazy

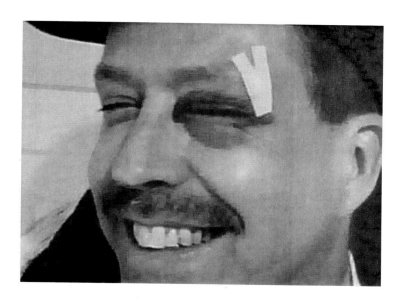

Dad's black eye

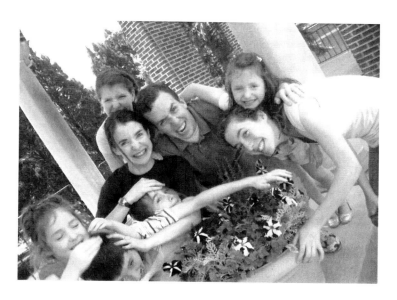

Very crazy

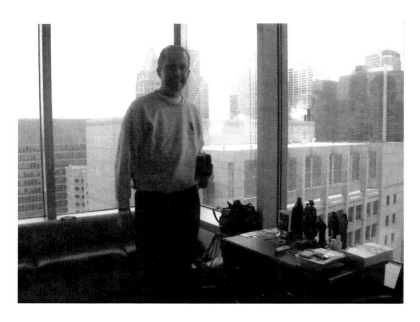

Jim in hospital room for bone marrow transplant

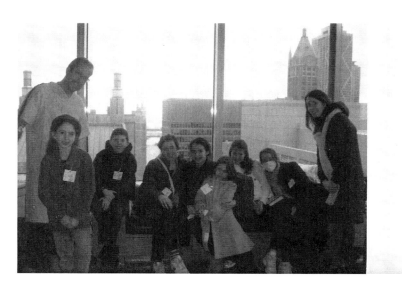

Children visiting in hospital

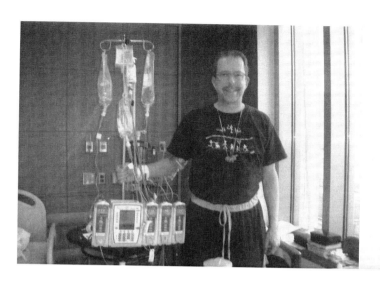

Jim posing with IVs. Are there enough

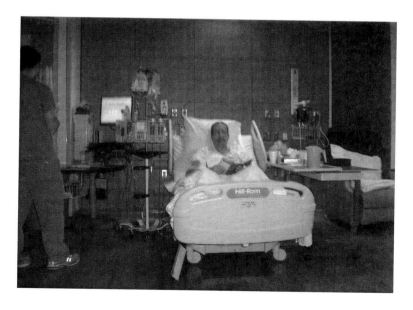

Jim praying scripture in hospital

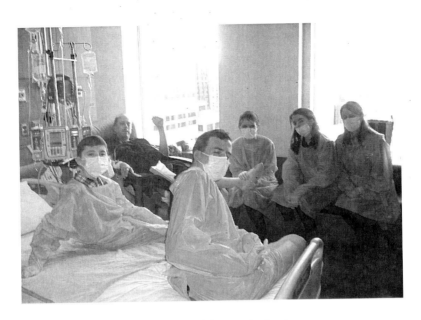

Visit in hospital by masked cohort

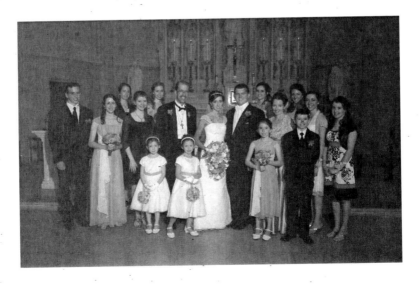

Family, Tara's Wedding

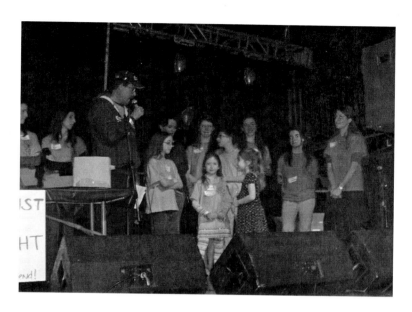

Jim addresses crowd at his benefit

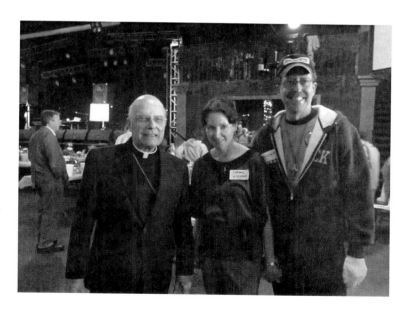

Francis Cardinal George with Jim & Kathleen at Benefit

179

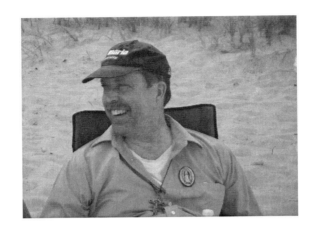

Jim at beach July 2012

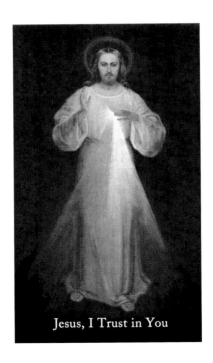

Jesus, I Trust in You

Divine Mercy Painting of Jesus

HEALING
IN THE GIFT OF LIFE

"I have set before you life and death, the blessing and the curse. Choose life, then, that you and your descendants may live" (Deuteronomy 30:19).

> Excerpt from my diary: September 16, 2010: Today I visited the graves of our miscarried children, Theresa Gerard, James Paul, and Frances Xavier. I prayed to all five of our miscarried children including Maximilian Mary and Joseph Faustina. I recommended the book I am attempting to write, *Healed through Cancer*, to their intercession. I prayed to and for them, and for my grandparents, Francis and Helen Littleton, at their graves. On the way home I noticed that there were slight parts in the clouds at various locations in the sky with very visible rays of white light shining down. I had the impression that, through my miscarried children's intercession, God was showering many graces down. Thanks be to God.

Kathleen and I have been blessed in our marriage with nineteen children ages twenty-five to five. Starting with the oldest they are: Shannon Rose, Tara Kathleen, Grace Ellen, Colleen Anne, Deirdre Marie, Bridget Jane, Shane Francis, Fiona Mary, Maura

Therese, Clare Margaret, Patrick Michael, Mairead Siobhan, Brighde Rosemarie, Shealagh Maeve; and our miscarried and still born children are: Maximilian Mary, Theresa Gerard, James Paul, Frances Xavier, and Joseph Faustina.

Interestingly, Kathleen had our first child at the age of twenty-six, and nine of our children, including six live births and three miscarriages, between the ages of thirty-eight and forty-six. Kathleen and I had experienced our fourth and fifth early miscarriages, Frances Xavier and Joseph Faustina, when Kathleen and I were in our early- to midforties. Then in our Bountiful Father's perfect plan came two more healthy babies, Brighde Rosemarie and, almost exactly one year later, when Kathleen was forty-six years old and I was forty-seven, Shealagh Maeve, our fourteenth living child and our nineteenth all together, counting our five babies in heaven.

We are truly an ordinary family. The trouble is that in this day and age an ordinary family has become extraordinary. May today's extraordinary become ordinary once again.

I am unapologetically *pro-choice*. I am using the morally correct definition of this term which means *pro-life*. I *choose* the truth—that is, to choose to do what is right and defend life at every time and in every way from the moment of conception until natural death. God invites and implores us to always choose life, though He will never force us, as He will never interfere with the gift of free will He has given to us.

Among other pro-life truths, I am totally opposed to abortion. Having said this, I do not condemn anyone who has had an abortion. I am opposed to the decision and the act. I leave judgment of the individual to God, whose bountiful mercy is always available when we repent. Kathleen and I are potentially guilty of abortion ourselves in that we used the *Pill* for a period of time before we started our family. We long ago repented of and regret this objectively grave sin, which has been washed away in the Precious Blood of our merciful Jesus.

The Pill does have an abortifacient property wherein break-through fertilization may occur while, at the same time, the Pill has made the lining of the womb (the endometrium) hostile toward the implantation of the fertilized egg—indeed a very small, unique, gifted, unrepeatable human being—thus causing the death of the baby.[42] Some may argue that there is not a human life present; but if there is not a human life, what in the world is it? The Church teaches the truth that life begins at conception, which is further defined as fertilization. At that moment, when the sperm fertilizes the egg, God infuses an immortal soul into the child. "Before I formed you in the womb I knew you; before you came to birth I consecrated you" (Jeremiah 1:5, JB). And no matter how small, the life of the child is just as important as any other. Can we ever justly base the value of a human being on his or her size, or some other nonessential attribute? Is a thirty-year-old, two-hundred pound, well-educated, affluent man more valuable than a one-year-old toddler? Of course not!

I had a sense that God, in the process of my illness, might give me the opportunity to stand up for my faith, pro-life convictions, and the objective moral truth. I imagined it might come in the form of some available treatment or medication involving embryonic stem cells obtained through the destruction of an embryo (a beautiful, unrepeatable, beloved child of God created with an immortal soul with an irreplaceable mission on earth). I would have to morally reject such treatment, no matter what the potential benefits for me. A basic, objective moral principle is that one cannot do evil that good may come of it. But our Blessed Father in heaven had a slightly different plan. His way is always the best.

I was very interested in a clinical trial at a teaching-university medical center involving a promising new drug, CAL 101. In the consent/disclosure form there was a portion to sign promising to use "birth control" to prevent pregnancy because of the potential danger of this drug to a child in the womb. I thought about this. I could morally agree to use Natural Family Planning (NFP), which is in a sense a form of "birth control," although I think, regardless, it is highly unlikely that Kathleen, age fifty-one, would get pregnant at this time since we had been open to life for the past five-and-a-half years without her becoming pregnant.

It occurred to me, however, that if I were to sign this consent/disclosure form, it would be culturally understood by the term "birth control" that I was agreeing to use immoral artificial forms of birth control contrary to the truth in regard to faith and morals as taught by the Catholic Church. This would be a scandal to others.

> Fecundity is a gift, an *end of marriage*, for conjugal love naturally tends to be fruitful. A child does not come from outside as something added on to the mutual love of the spouses, but springs from the very heart of that mutual giving, as its fruit and fulfillment. So the Church, which "is on the side of life,"[43] teaches that "it is necessary that each and every marriage act must remain open *per se* to the procreation of human life."[44] "This particular doctrine, expounded on numerous occasions by the Magisterium, is based on the inseparable connection, established by God, which man on his own initiative may not break, between the unitive significance and the procreative significance which are both inherent to the marriage act."[45]

> CCC 2366

In other words, each marital act must include both the element of unity, oneness, and pleasure along with the potential life-giving side of the act. This calls for openness to the gift of life and trust in God's providence.

Therefore, I had to qualify this point in accord with my beliefs in line with Church teaching. I left a message for the research coordinator indicating that I could not, in good conscience, use artificial birth control, which would be contrary to my beliefs in regard to faith and morals, but that we could use Natural Family Planning abstinence during fertile times, which is highly effective in postponing pregnancy when there is a just reason. We believed we had a just and even compelling reason to postpone having more children, if God so wished to gift us, with this life-and-death matter at hand.

> A particular aspect of this responsibility concerns the *regulation of procreation*. For just reasons, spouses may wish to space the births of their children. It is their duty to make certain that their desire is not motivated by selfishness but is in conformity with the generosity appropriate to responsible parenthood. Moreover, they should conform their behavior to the objective criteria of morality...
>
> CCC 2368

Regarding Natural Family Planning, which the Catholic Church endorses, and which I was proposing in lieu of means of artificial birth control:

> Periodic continence, that is, the methods of birth regulation based on self-observation and the use of infertile periods, is in conformity with the objective criteria of morality.[46] These methods respect the bodies of the spouses, encourage tenderness between them, and favor the education of an authentic freedom. In contrast, "every action which, whether in anticipation of the conjugal act, or in its accomplishment, or in the development of its natural consequences, proposes, whether as an end or as a means, to render procreation impossible" is intrinsically evil:[47]
>
> "Thus the innate language that expresses the total reciprocal self-giving of husband and wife is overlaid,

through contraception, by an objectively contradictory language, namely, that of not giving oneself totally to the other. This leads not only to a positive refusal to be open to life but also to a falsification of the inner truth of conjugal love, which is called upon to give itself in personal totality....The difference, both anthropological and moral, between contraception and recourse to the rhythm of the cycle...involves in the final analysis two irreconcilable concepts of the human person and of human sexuality."[48]

CCC 2370

I heard from the nurse later in the day indicating that the doctor was checking with the pharmaceutical company to see if they would allow me to participate in the study in consideration of my refusal to use artificial birth control. She seemed to express doubt that I would be accepted. I pointed out that Natural Family Planning is arguably more (and at least equally) effective than artificial means of birth control. I also pointed out that Kathleen is age fifty-one and unlikely to conceive regardless. I told her that under no circumstances could I use artificial birth control even if it were to mean my death the following day. This should not be considered either heroism or hyperbole. It is merely a duty that I must fulfill out of love for God, in spite of my very real human weakness and fears.

I sent some links regarding the effectiveness of NFP to the doctor who was the principal investigator with the trial.[49] She responded that she was trying to get in touch with the pharmaceutical company for a decision, and that they would perhaps have us sign a waiver of some sort so they would not be responsible in the event my wife, Kathleen, were to become pregnant and there was resulting damage done to the health of an unborn baby. I thought this would be fine.

I consider myself privileged to stand up for my faith in this way. It was really not difficult. "What profit would there be for one to gain the whole world and forfeit his life?" (Matthew 16:26). I was also inspired by the elderly man, Eleazar, in 2 Maccabees 6:18–31, who refused, at the cost of his life, even to give the pretense of eating pork (of sinning) because of the scandal it would cause others: "Just before he died under the blows, he groaned aloud and said, 'The Lord whose knowledge is holy sees clearly that, though I might have escaped death, whatever agonies of body I now endure under this bludgeoning, in my soul I am glad to suffer, because of the awe which he inspires in me'" (2 Maccabees 6:30, JB).

It is my privilege to be persecuted for the faith in any way, while at the same time I find it unjust to deny my access to this treatment because of my religious beliefs. Any such discrimination is unscientific in regard to Natural Family Planning as well, as it is a highly effective means of postponing pregnancy for a just reason.

> Edited excerpt from my diary: August 23, 2010: While I was in the chapel a phone message came in. After my hour of Eucharistic adoration I checked it, and it was the doctor/principal investigator stating that I was not going to be accepted in the clinical trial due to my refusal to use artificial birth control. I thank the Lord for the privilege of having an opportunity to—and for the grace of being willing and able to—stand up for my faith in this regard, as I had wanted to participate in this clinical trial a great deal. I accept God's will, which will bring a great good out of this injustice. I e-mailed the doctor and pointed out that there are over one billion Catholics in the world, and none of them can use artificial birth control in good conscience. Earlier I pointed out that the inclusion criteria of the study should allow for Natural Family Planning which is proven to be as effective as artificial means of contraception.

The doctor had also mentioned complete abstinence as an option, but that would be totally unnecessary and oppressive considering that the use of the trial drug could go on for many years. Since there is the alleged and apparently unproven risk of harm to an unborn child through the use of this drug, I could have, in good conscience, agreed to practice Natural Family Planning to avoid conception during fertile times; though, quite honestly, considering the *negligible* risk, I would have preferred to be open to life and leave the outcome in God's good hands, as any life conceived is a good life. Only God knows whether a child would be born healthy or not, and an "unhealthy" child certainly has as much value as a healthy child.

It is interesting that on the day I was notified that I would not be accepted in the trial, the themes of justice and truthfulness kept coming up in my prayer meditations—truthfulness in the sense that even a small lie or deception must be avoided. Though I could have signed this disclosure knowing that "birth control" includes Natural Family Planning, there would have been deception involved, as the writer of the document certainly intended *artificial* birth control, the cultural definition. There is also the concern about scandal to others wherein they would think that I was willing to use artificial birth control in order to take this new drug for my cancer.

I ran into the same scenario with another clinical trial I had been interested in where I was also denied treatment for the same reasons. That case was decided by the Institutional Review Board (IRB). This injustice is clearly systemic to the medical community.

At any rate, I have since undergone a stem-cell transplant, which may turn out to have been the best possible treatment choice, though I did not think that at the time I was pursuing the clinical trials. Well, "God knows how to write straight with crooked lines."[50]

I was privileged to have God permit me to be in a position to live my faith by making a potentially costly choice to *walk the talk* of what I believe, and try my best to live it with all my heart and soul. This was accomplished only by the aid of His grace. Though I was fearful on a human level of what this would mean to my life and health, I can honestly say that I did experience a profound peace and joy deep in my soul over being given and sustained through this opportunity to show my love for Jesus and my neighbor.

God has endowed us with the power to cocreate life utilizing our gift of sexuality. This is another power that makes us much like Him, through no merit of our own. It is purely a gift. As the Love between the Father and the Son bears fruit as the third Person (namely, the Holy Spirit) of the Most Holy Trinity, three divine persons, one God, so does the love between man and wife bear fruit in the third person of a beautiful child. Husband and wife are called to hold nothing back from the other, to surrender everything, to die to themselves in giving all they are and have to the other, as Jesus prayed to His Father: "All I have is yours and all you have is mine" (John 17:10, JB). True love between husband and wife is called to be entirely reciprocal, not holding back, especially in our God-given gift and power of fertility.

Jesus Christ and His Church have raised sex above the banal pursuit of pleasure to a sacrament, or something sacred. Each time a married couple unites in one flesh they are renewing their marriage vows, in a sense dying to themselves, so as to give themselves completely to each other. Some translations of holy Scripture read: "And Adam knew Eve his wife; and she conceived" (Genesis 4:1, King James Bible). When man and wife become one flesh they truly come to *know* the other in the most profound way possible. This special knowing is only for them, no one else; thus absolute fidelity is expected and vowed to by the spouses when they enter into matrimony. There needs to be a lifelong indissoluble commitment for such a splendid gift to be shared.

Sexual activity, properly engaged in between husband and wife, is sacred and respects the dignity of the other, who is a temple of the Holy Spirit. What we do with our body, we also do with our soul and spirit, which are all inseparable. It is not as if the soul is isolated and hidden away somewhere such as in the heart. No, it permeates the entire body. Our bodies too are sacred, as are the bodies of others. Our bodies are not even our own property. We have been bought and paid for by our Lord Jesus. "Your body, you know, is the temple of the Holy Spirit, who is in you since you received him from God. You are not your own property; you have been bought and paid for. That is why you should use your body for the glory of God" (1 Corinthians 6:19–20, JB). May we do everything for the glory of God!

Love is never selfish (see 1 Corinthians 13:4–5). Our sexuality is not something to be squandered or demeaned with a multiplicity of people. We should never make objects of others for our own pleasure. Thus, pornography is always wrong and disordered. With pornography one takes pleasure at the expense of the degradation of others. "Love takes no pleasure in other people's sins but delights in the truth" (1 Corinthians 13:6, JB).

Unfortunately there is an epidemic of pornography today. Many are addicted. And as with any addiction the assistance of a Higher Power is needed in order to break with it.

I think that the Church's teaching on the truth and magnificence of human sexuality is easier to comprehend when one has a heavy cross to carry like cancer, as we tend to become more open to the grace of God needed to understand, embrace, live, and persevere in these and other objectively true moral teachings. We are healed by God in that we receive a much greater capacity to comprehend the truth about how precious every life truly is, as we experience in a critical way the fragility of our own precious life.

Never fear. God is with us to show the way, and to give us all the help we need to live true love. But we cannot live this without Him.

I would like to conclude this chapter with a ballad I wrote many years ago in adoration before Jesus in the Blessed Sacrament. I pray that it not only depicts the real tragedy of abortion, but also Jesus's love and available forgiveness and mercy for those responsible.

FAREWELL OF THE UNBORN MARTYR[51]

1

The struggle is over, I have been defeated
The room here is covered with evil and gloom
An unborn child in the womb of my mother
A nurse and a doctor plan to tear me apart
No crime was committed but my sentence is murder
My mother lies scared and in terrible pain
My father is outside, he will not defend me
No friends have I here, but some dear souls outside

CHORUS:

Love for my parents I carry in my heart
I lay down my life for my Mom and my Dad
Farewell to this world God willed me to live in
In love have I lived, and a martyr I'll die (I've died)

2

My dreams have been broken, my plans have been shattered
No birthdays or cakes, no schoolbooks for me
I will not get married, or have any children
But the love which I have will never be spent

For the instruments seek me, they will tear my body
As I carry my cross as my Lord did before
The pain from the cutting is excruciating
But this does not compare with my abandonment

3

No name was I given by my parents who forsake me
I'll await their conversion while I behold God's Face
Someday they will name me when blessed with true sorrow
God waits with forgiveness through the Love of Jesus
Who was innocent when He gave up His Body
And Blood on the Cross so that we may all live
My Baptism comes by the blood of my torture
My Christening gown is the womb of my mom

4

I did receive some love on the morning of my death
Some souls who did care were out praying for me
A rosary they gave to my mother that morning
As she rushed by those watching and praying for us
My Dad only cursed them as he felt so guilty
My Mom threw the Rosary back down at their feet
If only they had listened to the prayers and the wisdom
How happy I'd be to have a chance at life

5

I now have been killed, my body is broken
The Mother of Jesus comes to carry me away
She holds me and rocks me while her tears fall on my face
Her tears are for me and my Mom and my Dad.

Mary brings me before my dear Father in Heaven
Along with my angel who kept watch over me
My Jesus receives me, the Holy Spirit fills me
While we all shed tears of love for my Mom and my Dad

HEALING THROUGH HUMILITY

"The greatest among you must be your servant. Whoever exalts himself will be humbled; but whoever humbles himself will be exalted" (Matthew 23:11–12). Here we see again that God's ways are not naturally our ways. We are called to be servants or slaves to others.

Humility is truth, the truth of who we are, including the good and bad. The truth is that we are beloved children of God, each of us, no one excluded. This is assured. The truth is also that God is God, and we are not. He is our creator and savior, and He is all knowing.

In constant battle with the virtue of humility is the ego or self. We have a tendency of being self-centered. I have found through experience that the best means of achieving humility is through humiliations and the cross, especially those that God arranges for us, which tend to cut the deepest into the hidden regions of our being where the ego hides. Humility is a key virtue. Other virtues are difficult if not impossible to acquire without a meaningful measure of humility.

If our cup is full of our ego and pride, then there is no room for God to fill it. If, with God's help, we empty our cup of self, then there is room for God to fill our cup with Himself and His virtues of faith, hope, love/charity, prudence, justice, temperance, and fortitude. "And from pride preserve your servant, never let it dominate me" (Psalm 19:13, JB).

For example, in my life, and perhaps yours, I have had to accept and even seek help from others at different times, especially during my illness. This is a cross and humiliation. I remember when my business was doing very well about twelve years ago and I was in the position of being able to help others with gifts of money. In retrospect this was much easier than humbling myself to receive gifts from others in my need. Though I willed and tried my best to give God the glory when I was in a position to help others, I felt powerful and self-sufficient having the means to give to others. It is much easier to give than to receive in this sense.

It can seem impossible to eradicate a disordered ego. It seems the best we can do is to knock it down time and again through whatever means we have available. It cannot be killed. It keeps coming back to rear its ugly head. The reality of our disordered ego is part of the battlefield of life where we have the opportunity to fight and gain merit.

Some of the means of keeping the disordered ego at bay include prayer, seeking God's readily available help, acceptance of crosses and humiliations, and focusing our lives on serving others. I have always noticed that the happiest people are those who are the most generous and giving of their time, talent, and treasures.

God accomplishes His greatest deeds through humble souls. The most humble person who ever lived, besides the God-man Jesus, was the Blessed Virgin Mary. She is the Model of Humility. "My soul proclaims the greatness of the Lord;/ my spirit rejoices in God my savior./ For he has looked upon his handmaid's lowliness;/ behold, from now on will all ages call me blessed./ The Mighty One has done great things for me,/ and holy is his name" (Luke 1:46–49).

Mary admits her lowliness. She then tells the truth that all ages will call her blessed, but she immediately gives the glory to God in truth. Mary was immaculately conceived, meaning she was born without sin and never sinned; however, she also suffered greater crosses and humiliations than any person ever born or ever to be born, other than Jesus Himself. The most painful type of suffering is interior suffering. Mary's interior suffering was immense including such events as the Holy Family's flight into Egypt, the Way of the Cross, and Jesus's crucifixion and burial.

The more innocent and pure a person is, the more he or she will suffer in the presence of evil. Mary was and is pure beyond our comprehension. Take an innocent ten-year-old child and expose him or her to Jesus's crucifixion while standing at the foot of the cross, and take a seasoned soldier who has seen many battles, casualties, and deaths. Who suffers the most? The innocent child, of course. This gives us a dim understanding of how much the Blessed Virgin Mary must have suffered. This suffering and humiliation only increased her humility, if it was possible for this virtue to increase in her, beyond its incomprehensive, already-exalted level.

Cancer and other heavy crosses heal us in that they are efficacious means of attaining the queen virtue of humility.

One of Jesus's final acts on His last evening before His death the following day was to wash the feet of His apostles. We look at John 13:4–5, 13–15:

> [Jesus] rose from supper and took off his outer garments. He took a towel and tied it around his waist. Then he poured water into a basin and began to wash the disciples' feet and dry them with the towel around his waist....
>
> "You call me 'teacher' and 'master,' and rightly so, for indeed I am. If I, therefore, the master and teacher, have washed your feet, you ought to wash one another's feet. I have given you a model to follow, so that as I have done for you, you should also do."

The apostles feet were likely very smelly, disgusting, and filthy after a hot day of walking in sandals through the dirt. To wash their feet was the dirty, humble work of a slave. Jesus was giving us an inspiring model to follow of humility and service. Let us follow the Master's example.

> Do nothing out of selfishness or out of vainglory; rather, humbly regard others as more important than yourselves, each looking out not for his own interests, but [also] everyone for those of others.
>
> Have among yourselves the same attitude that is also yours in Christ Jesus,/ Who, though he was in the form of God,/ did not regard equality with God/ something to be grasped./ Rather, he emptied himself,/ taking the form of a slave,/ coming in human likeness;/ and found human in appearance,/ he humbled himself,/ becoming obedient to death,/ even death on a cross./ Because of this, God greatly exalted him/ and bestowed on him the name/ that is above every name,/ that at the name of Jesus/ every knee should bend,/ of those in heaven and on earth and under the earth,/ and every tongue confess that/ Jesus Christ is Lord,/ to the glory of God the Father.
>
> Philippians 2:3–11

Yes, Jesus is Lord!

The following scripture, Job 33:16–30 (JB), seems to directly describe experiences I have gone through more than once in my illness, in many cases quite literally. Perhaps you will recognize your own experiences in this beautiful passage:

> Then it is he whispers in the ear of man, or may frighten him with fearful sights, to turn him away from evil-doing, and make an end of his pride; to save his soul from the

pit and his life from the pathway to Sheol. With suffering, too, he corrects man on his sick-bed, when his bones keep trembling with palsy; when his whole life is revolted by food, and his appetite spurns dainties; when his flesh rots as you watch it, and his bare bones begin to show; when his soul is drawing near to the pit, and his life to the dwelling of the dead. Then there is an Angel by his side, a Mediator, chosen out of thousands, to remind a man where his duty lies, to take pity on him and to say, "Release him from descent into the pit, for I have found a ransom for his life"; his flesh recovers the bloom of its youth, he lives again as he did when he was young. He prays to God who has restored him to favour, and comes, in happiness, to see his face. He publishes far and wide the news of his vindication, singing before his fellow men this hymn of praise, "I sinned and left the path of right, but God has not punished me as my sin deserved. He has spared my soul from going down into the pit, and is allowing my life to continue in the light." All this God does again and yet again for man, rescuing his soul from the pit, and letting the light of life shine bright on him.

I don't think this passage needs much commentary. Note that the sufferings are meant to help the soul to grow in the virtue of humility, to overcome his pride, and to save his soul. We note that in this case God saves when things appear to be at their worst. "For God everything is possible" (Matthew 19:26, JB) and all is designed to work out for our best according to God's plan, whatever the outcome, be it healing, including continuation of life here on earth, or death leading to the resurrection. Let us be happy, for God is revealing His Face to us. A ransom has been found for our life, the sacrifice and death of our Blessed Lord, Jesus!

We have been given so many healings and gifts from our Heavenly Father. We must share these blessing and songs of hope with others who are so desperately in need. We are called to be humble, grateful people unabashedly publishing far and wide the news of our vindication, singing before our fellow men our *hymn of praise.*

We are called to use our free will to permit God to circumcise our hearts, transforming them into hearts of love. "Circumcise your heart then and be obstinate no longer" (Deuteronomy 10:16–17, JB). In His perfect, loving providence God will often permit a cross in our life so that our hearts might be healed. "I in my turn will set myself against them and take them to the land of their enemies. Then their uncircumcised heart will be humbled, then they will atone for their sins. I shall remember my Covenant with Jacob, and my Covenant with Isaac and my Covenant with Abraham; and I shall remember the land" (Leviticus 26:41–42, JB).

It is the Humble and Sacred Heart of Jesus that heals us, humbles us, and creates a new heart for us. "The real circumcision is in the heart—something not of the letter but of the spirit" (Romans 2:29, JB).

HEALING THROUGH MERCY AND FORGIVENESS

"But to you who hear I say, love your enemies, do good to those who hate you, bless those who curse you, pray for those who mistreat you. To the person who strikes you on one cheek, offer the other one as well, and from the person who takes your cloak, do not withhold even your tunic. Give to everyone who asks of you, and from the one who takes what is yours do not demand it back. Do to others as you would have them do to you. For if you love those who love you, what credit is that to you? Even sinners love those who love them. And if you do good to those who do good to you, what credit is that to you? Even sinners do the same. If you lend money to those from whom you expect repayment, what credit [is] that to you? Even sinners lend to sinners, and get back the same amount. But rather, love your enemies and do good to them, and lend expecting nothing back; then your reward will be great and you will be children of the Most High, for he himself is kind to the ungrateful and the wicked. Be merciful, just as [also] your Father is merciful.

"Stop judging and you will not be judged. Stop condemning and you will not be condemned. Forgive and you will be forgiven. Give and gifts will be given to you; a good measure, packed together, shaken down, and overflowing, will be poured into your lap. For the measure with which you measure will in return be measured out to you."

Luke 6:27–38

Mercy and forgiveness go both ways, God toward us, and us toward others. As far as others forgiving us, we cannot control that. It is a futile waste of time and energy to try to control others. We can only control, with the help of God's grace, our own attitudes and actions.

In Matthew 18:23–35 you find the parable of the "king who decided to settle accounts with his servants. When he began the accounting, a debtor was brought before him who owed him a huge amount. Since he had no way of paying it back, his master ordered him to be sold, along with his wife, his children, and all his property, in payment of the debt." This is depicted in some translations as an amount essentially so huge it could never hope to be paid back. This represents our debt to God. When we sin we offend the infinite, which creates an infinite debt. Being finite we can never repay that debt ourselves.

An offence is always greater as it relates to the status of the person offended. If I strike a friend in a dispute, the penalty under the law will not be nearly as great as it would be if I struck the president of the United States. Therefore our infinite God, Jesus, became man in order to take our place upon the cross in His passion and death so as to satisfy the infinite debt we brought upon ourselves with our sins. How does our Heavenly Father treat us? With infinite mercy! We all need and want mercy, and it is readily available for us from our loving Eternal Father.

It is true that God holds the keys to the Kingdom of Heaven, and thanks be to God, He shares these keys with Peter, the Pope, the head of His merciful Church here on earth. What else does the Church primarily exist for other than to be the fount and dispenser of the infinite mercy of Jesus? "So I now say to you: You are Peter and on this rock I will build my Church. And the gates of the underworld can never hold out against it. I will give you the keys of the kingdom of heaven" (Matthew 16:18–19, JB). And hear this! By His passion, death, and resurrection, Jesus has given each of us the keys to His merciful heart, which poured forth for us water and blood, the Sacraments of Baptism and Eucharist, His very Holy Spirit of Love, His Divine Life! "One of the soldiers pierced his side with a lance; and immediately there came out blood and water" (John 19:34–35, JB).

We are a broken, sinful, fearful, wounded people. We do not have the power to save ourselves, and bring ourselves to eternal life in heaven. We need only repent to receive God's abundant mercy. Repentance is liberating. We are honest with ourselves, and admit to our dependency on God. Jesus came to "set free all those who had been held in slavery all their lives by the fear of death" (Hebrews 2:15, JB).

Returning to Matthew 18:23–35: "At that, the servant fell down, did him homage, and said, 'Be patient with me, and I will pay you back in full.' Moved with compassion the master of the servant let him go and forgave him the loan. When that servant had left, he found one of his fellow servants who owed him a much smaller amount." Our offences against each other are finite regardless of their level of seriousness. We are called to have compassion on and forgive others, as God has compassion on and forgives us.

"He seized him and started to choke him, demanding, 'Pay back what you owe.' Falling to his knees, his fellow servant begged him, 'Be patient with me, and I will pay you back.'" Yes, be patient—this is what we are called to be with each other, to be merciful and forgiving.

"But he refused. Instead, he had him put in prison until he paid back the debt." We can clearly grasp the injustice in the lack of forgiveness here when the debtor who had been forgiven an impossibly huge amount refused to forgive his fellow servant a comparatively small sum, mercilessly holding a grudge, demanding restitution, venting his rage and bitterness, and choking him.

"Now when his fellow servants saw what had happened, they were deeply disturbed, and went to their master and reported the whole affair." Do we not often become disturbed when we encounter injustice involving others? Yet we tend to be slow in noticing our own unjust actions.

"His master summoned him and said to him, 'You wicked servant! I forgave you your entire debt because you begged me to. Should you not have had pity on your fellow servant, as I had pity on you?' Then in anger his master handed him over to the torturers until he should pay back the whole debt. So will my heavenly Father do to you unless each of you forgives his brother from his heart."

Yes, it can be very costly, but we have the irrefutable obligation to forgive everything in a heartfelt way. This is a primary condition of our receiving mercy. This forgiveness should be immediate and with no limit on the number of times we forgive. "Then Peter approaching asked him, 'Lord, if my brother sins against me, how often must I forgive him? As many as seven times?' Jesus answered, 'I say to you, not seven times but seventy-seven times'" (Matthew 18:21–22).

Who and what must we forgive? Everyone and everything. Are there any exceptions? No! Is there any offense exempt from our forgiveness? No! None? No! Why? Because God stands ready to forgive anyone and everyone for the worse imaginable sin, no exceptions, no matter how many times, if we only repent and accept that forgiveness. This is the essence of mercy. Mercy has no limits. God's mercy is infinite. We must strive to be people of mercy, to be perfect as our Heavenly Father is perfect. "So be perfect, just as your heavenly Father is perfect" (Matthew 5:48).

We release ourselves from bondage when we forgive and gain peace and happiness. This is dependent on us, not the person we are forgiving, even though that person may not give a rat's... behind that we are forgiving him or her.

This type of forgiveness is divine and takes more than we can muster on our own. We need the divine help of the Holy Spirit, which is readily available.

> So, then, I discover the principle that when I want to do right, evil is at hand. For I take delight in the law of God, in my inner self, but I see in my members another principle at war with the law of my mind, taking me captive to the law of sin that dwells in my members. Miserable one that I am! Who will deliver me from this mortal body? Thanks be to God through Jesus Christ our Lord. Therefore, I myself, with my mind, serve the law of God but, with my flesh, the law of sin.
>
> Romans 7:21–25

How can we be perfect? Only through grace. I believe that the need for forgiveness toward others is a major reason why we need a strong prayer life, and for Catholics first and foremost a consistent and deep sacramental life. We need the grace to rise above our fallen human nature, which is so quick to be unmerciful and hold on to grudges and bitterness. We tend to want to seize and *choke* the one who offended us. *He had him put in prison until he paid back the debt.* The one we really put in prison is our self when we refuse to forgive. When we have mercy we are freed.

We need grace in order to be transformed into Christ in whom we are gifted with the capacity to decide, although extremely difficult, to forgive others. This is a must. I am convinced that serious illness such as cancer heals us by providing us with the additional fortification we need to be a persons of mercy. Cancer and other serious illnesses and tragedies in life help us to come to know ourselves better, to recognize how imperfect and sinful we have been, to see the plank, or in my case the *railroad tie*, in our own eye, and to realize how needy we are of God's mercy. We are also healed in our understanding of how ready God is with His *healing balm* of forgiveness toward us, and how beloved we are by our Heavenly Father.

Luke 7:36–50: "A Pharisee invited him to dine with them, and he entered the Pharisee's house and reclined at table. Now there was a sinful woman in the city who learned he was at table in the house of the Pharisee." Are we not all sinners in need of God's mercy?

"Bringing an alabaster flask of ointment, she stood behind him at his feet weeping and began to bathe his feet with her tears. She then wiped them with her hair, kissed them, and anointed them with the ointment." Our sentiments and tears of love and sorrow for our failings are truly an *ointment that consoles* the Heart of our Lord Jesus.

"When the Pharisee who had invited him saw this he said to himself, 'If this man were a prophet, he would know who and what sort of woman this is who is touching him, that she is a sinner.'" May we all be healed from our tendency to judge others. Only God knows and understands the complex tapestry of each individual's life including his or her culpability or lack thereof. Besides, we have a lifetime of tough work ahead of us surmounting our own imperfections by pushing them out with our growth in virtue. And how did the Pharisee know the type of woman this was anyway?[52] What was his history of contribution toward her "sinfulness"? Did he check the plank in his own eye before condemning this contrite woman, who stood very much higher in Jesus's eyes than he did? Yes, Jesus most certainly was a Prophet, the Source of all true prophets! He knew who in the room was the person most in need of conversion, and it wasn't the woman!

How does Jesus answer? With one of His parables, of course. The beauty of parables is that each contains an infinity of helpful, truthful nuances, as well as divine guidance for the reader, since they are the Word of God. "Jesus said to him in reply, 'Simon, I have something to say to you.'" And we should reply to Jesus as did the Pharisee, as cancer helps reveal to us that we all have some bit of a Pharisee in us that needs to be purged and healed. "Tell me, teacher." When You speak, Lord Jesus, please give us the grace to listen! "'Two people were in debt to a certain creditor; one owed five hundred days' wages and the other owed fifty. Since they were unable to repay the debt, he forgave it for both. Which of them will love him more?' Simon said in reply, 'The one, I suppose, whose larger debt was forgiven.' He said to him, 'You have judged rightly.'" We all have debts that need to be brought to Jesus so that they may be readily forgiven, some larger and some smaller, but all more than we can resolve on our own since we have indebted ourselves through sin against the Infinite. So we are all in the same boat so to speak, the *SS Sinner*.

"Then he turned to the woman and said to Simon, 'Do you see this woman?'" This is such a powerful statement: *Do you see this woman?* Do we really see our fellow man as he truly is, a beloved, unique, unrepeatable child of our Heavenly Father, a connected brother or sister, weighed down with countless troubles, and desiring Perfect Love just as we do? Or do we see our neighbors as objects or obstacles? Cancer is a powerful means of helping us to see our neighbor as Jesus sees him or her, with compassion, mercy, empathy, and deep love.

> When I entered your house, you did not give me water for my feet, but she has bathed them with her tears and wiped them with her hair. You did not give me a kiss, but she has

not ceased kissing my feet since the time I entered. You did not anoint my head with oil, but she anointed my feet with ointment. So I tell you, her many sins have been forgiven; hence, she has shown great love. But the one to whom little is forgiven, loves little.

Here is another example of God's ways not being our ways, how His ways are, as a rule, 180 degrees reverse of our ways. Here He is telling us that one who was the greater sinner is now the greater lover. What love and hope this inspires! This passage has personally given me immense consolation and hope over the years because I have been such a great sinner.

I have also experienced Jesus's awesome mercy and have, at least to a degree, been enabled to be more compassionate and to understand others where they are at. I want to lift everyone up to Jesus! And His unconditional mercy toward me and my innumerable sins moves me to be immensely grateful and to love Him all the more.

"He said to her, 'Your sins are forgiven.'" What incredible peace these words bring when they are spoken by Christ! Yes, Jesus is merciful, and "God's love endures forever" (Psalm 136:1), toward everyone who will accept it. But, for those of us who have been blessed with the gift of a vibrant Catholic faith, we have the special gift and peace of hearing these words spoken audibly to us by Christ through the mouth of the priest, *in persona Christi* (meaning in the person of Christ), after each participation in the Sacrament of Confession (also known as Penance and Reconciliation):

God the Father of mercies, through the death and resurrection of his Son, has reconciled the world to himself and sent the Holy Spirit among us for the forgiveness of sins; through the ministry of the Church may God give you pardon and peace, and I absolve you from your sins in the name of the Father, and of the Son, and of the Holy Spirit. [53]

CCC 1449

Oh what peace and joy won by the Blood of Christ are given to us in each confession!

Note the words of Jesus to St. Faustina recorded in her Diary:

> Write, speak of My mercy. Tell souls where they are to look for solace; that is, in the Tribunal of Mercy [the Sacrament of Reconciliation also known as Confession]. There the greatest miracles take place [and] are incessantly repeated. To avail oneself of this miracle, it is not necessary to go on a great pilgrimage or to carry out some external ceremony; it suffices to come with faith to the feet of My representative and to reveal to him one's misery, and the miracle of Divine Mercy will be fully demonstrated. Were a soul like a decaying corpse so that from a human standpoint, there would be no [hope of] restoration and everything would already be lost, it is not so with God. The miracle of Divine Mercy restores that soul in full. Oh, how miserable are those who do not take advantage of the miracle of God's mercy! You will call out in vain, but it will be too late.

Diary 1448[54]

May we never despair. Mercy is always available. We need only take advantage of the opportunity to admit our misery and take advantage of this awesome gift while we live and the opportunity exists.

What was Christ's worst suffering when carrying the cross? The answer is that His cross was too light, because of those sins He foresaw would not be placed on His cross, because of those souls who would be lost for refusing to accept the gift of His mercy. Mystically, I believe that is why He struggled and fell. This was His worse suffering, to realize that His incredible redemptive act of suffering and death would be wasted in its application to certain souls! Oh, how He loves souls! He could not bear the pain that some might be lost. All sins placed on Christ's cross obtain His mercy. All sins that we retain on our own back will simply crush us. What sins are we still carrying on our back? Console Christ! He wants the extra weight of our sins off our backs and onto *His*! This will make Him enormously pleased.

Perhaps one thinks that a particular sin or sins are unforgivable, such as the unforgivable sin against the Holy Spirit mentioned in the gospel. Yes, it is true, there is one unforgiveable sin. That sin is the one we choose not to repent of. Every sin is forgivable, and by "every" we mean *every* sin! This is not just my opinion, but Jesus Himself speaking through His Church as to proper interpretation of Scripture.

> "Therefore I tell you, every sin and blasphemy will be forgiven men, but the blasphemy against the Spirit will not be forgiven."[55] There are no limits to the mercy of God, but anyone who deliberately refuses to accept his mercy by repenting, rejects the forgiveness of his sins and the salvation offered by the Holy Spirit.[56] Such hardness of heart can lead to final impenitence and eternal loss.
>
> CCC 1864

What sins of ours do we think could possibly be too heavy for our infinitely strong God? Let's not be foolish and proud! Come to His infinite mercy!

How much does Jesus love us? He chose to bear the scars on His hands, feet, and side into heaven. I believe He is constantly showing His wounds to His Father saying, "See how much I love them!" He tells us through His prophet, "See, I have branded you on the palms of my hands" (Isaiah 49:16, JB). When Jesus looks at His hands, He looks at us through the holes with unimaginable love! How inexpressibly happy He is when we take advantage of His mercy, won at so high a price!

What is God's will? Our Heavenly Father's will holds His mercy. His infinite mercy is His infinite will. If we desire mercy, we must throw ourselves into the abyss of His will, which will involve suffering and purification, and where we will encounter mercy in the person of Christ. In this abyss of sorrow and joy, mysteriously mixed, we will receive mercy, and be conformed into the image of His Son, Jesus, so that we will become ladles in His hand for dispensing mercy to other souls.

HEALING IN ACCEPTING MYSELF

"Do not be afraid, Jacob, poor worm, Israel, puny mite. I will help you—it is Yahweh who speaks—the Holy One of Israel is your redeemer" (Isaiah 41:14, JB).

Humility is truth. It is reality. God is God. I am not. It is a highly beneficial exercise to reflect on myself to come to know myself better, including all that is good, bad, and ugly. I believe another way God heals us through a heavy cross is that we become more able and willing to know ourselves in truth, and then to hopefully accept ourselves. I know by life experience, especially since my illness, that it is true that I am the *puny mite* referred to by God in the above passage. Yet, He tells me not to be afraid! He is helping me each step of the way. He is my redeemer!

I do not possess anything that is not a gift from God including my very life, as well as all my talents and possessions. "What do you have that was not given to you? And if it was given, how can you boast as though it were not?" (1 Corinthians 4: 7–8, JB). I am totally dependent on Him for everything.

Is there good in each of us? Yes, enormous good. God only makes masterpieces! He does not make mistakes. God has given each of us inimitable gifts and a unique mission that only we can fulfill.

Are all of us sinners? Yes, join the club. Part of knowing oneself is the painful process of admitting one's faults, sins, and weaknesses. "If we say we have no sin in us, we are deceiving ourselves and refusing to admit the truth; but if we acknowledge our sins, then God who is faithful and just will forgive our sins and purify us from everything that is wrong" (1 John 1:8–9, JB).

I am not saying that we have a license to sin and that sin is not a concern. Sin does offend God, and it hurts others. Most of all it hurts ourselves. But when sin happens, we should not be dispirited but quickly and confidently repent and turn to God for His inexhaustible mercy. Not until we admit our shortcomings can we begin to improve ourselves with God's always available help.

When we repent and convert we are healed. It takes just an effort on our part. God faithfully does the rest. We are enlightened by the Holy Spirit; we begin to open our eyes and take the earplugs out, so as to begin to see and hear again the truth about ourselves and about God. "You will listen and listen again, but not understand, see and see again, but not perceive. For the heart of this nation has grown coarse, their ears are dull of hearing, and they have shut their eyes, for fear they should see with their eyes, hear with their ears, understand with their heart, and be converted and healed by me" (Matthew 13:14–15, JB).

It is no use being afraid to see ourselves in the light of God. We can't hide anything. He already knows us inside and out, infinitely better than we know ourselves. Truly profound self-knowledge and understanding is a gift that only God can give. It is available for the asking. We need simply to knock at God's door. "The one who knocks will always have the door opened to him" (Matthew 7:8, JB). Yes, it will be painful seeing our faults and sins, but we need to acknowledge that we are sinners and repent so that the rivers of God's mercy may be allowed to run free, and so that we will receive true peace.

We are all called to the battle of growing in virtue. This is a battle where there are many falls. This battle will never end until our last breath. We need to put the archenemy of discouragement to the sword, and keep picking ourselves up again. We need to accept ourselves, the ostensible wreck we may be in many ways, and decide to love ourselves as God loves us: unconditionally. Admittedly this can be very difficult to do, but God's help will never be lacking if we ask.

When we are too hard on ourselves we can tend to be too hard on others. I know this by experience. I think we need to be merciful with ourselves if we are to be entirely merciful with others.

Anything good in me comes from God. Anything bad is my own doing. I know that regardless of our faults, weaknesses, and limitations God sees each of us as His masterpiece in the works. "My grace is enough for you: my power is at its best in weakness" (2 Corinthians 12:9, JB). We must rely on the power of Jesus, not our own supposed power. He is the potter, we the clay. "And yet, Yahweh, you are our Father; we the clay, you the potter, we are all the work of your hand" (Isaiah 64:8, JB). It comes down to this: we are all beloved children of our Merciful Father in heaven, and we are all in need of His help for everything, no exceptions—most especially needing His readily available mercy so that we might be happy with Him for all eternity.

I personally need to accept that I can be a cross to others, and often am. Part of the reason for this is that the human body weighs me down (though I admit a copious degree of fault on my part and that I am very much in need of Jesus's mercy). I have many ups and downs in the way I act, especially toward those I love the most: my own wife and children.

Probably the biggest way I am a cross to others, most especially to my family who has to live with me, is in the effects of my obsessive-compulsive behavior. This is a major cross to me, and it is a cross to them. This contributes to my being extremely demanding and impatient, often over the most negligible things. I am very sorry that my family has had to suffer from this.

My obsessive-compulsive disorder (OCD) is very much a disorder that brings much pain with it like any disease. However, like with all things God permits, there has been a positive side to it, because He is always mysteriously bringing good out of everything. Because of it in part I have perhaps had the extra drive to accomplish many good things such as being an entrepreneur (though not a very good one) and writing this book (I hope this book is a good thing). It also gives me a battlefield on which to gain greater merit in my efforts to be patient, which is all the more challenging, though I admit that I do not try nearly as hard as I should. Sometimes I can be very virtuous. Others times I can behave dreadfully, ashamedly poorly.

I am a weak human being struggling with my cross as you are with yours; even Jesus was not exactly jolly on the cross, because it was hard beyond comprehension. For those of us who are suffering from cancer or some other serious illness it is good to keep in mind that we are composed of spirit, soul, and body. It is hard on us. It is okay if we handle this monumental challenge in a less than perfect way. We are human. When the body ails it affects everything. "He knows what we are made of" (Psalm 103:14, JB).

Don't be too hard on yourself. What would you think if it was your child who had cancer and was testy and down in spirit at times? Wouldn't you understand? Wouldn't you love her all the more? Well, God our Father is infinite love and mercy, and I am certain He is actually very proud of you.

It is encouraging to remember this reality that you can count on: your prayers and suffering are worth more than ever principally when things are hardest and darkest, when you struggle the most. Keep uniting them with confidence to Jesus. As difficult as it may be to comprehend, be assured that through these things, God is bringing great benefit to you and others. And this is giving glory to God our Father who so loves His children. Jesus, I trust in You!

Keep hoping. Keep living life to the full. You are alive today. This is a gem to be celebrated and lived to the full. You are full of life. You have a tremendous capacity to do so much good, as I know you have been doing. Do everything out of love. Never fear. Only trust. Keep making that act of the will. Jesus, I trust in You! There are many praying for you. May you live many more years, but whenever the Lord Jesus decides to take you to heaven, you will be amazed and so pleased for all eternity at how many other people are there, or on their way, thanks to your life of prayer, service, and the cross.

HEALING IN ACCEPTING OTHERS

"We who are strong ought to put up with the failings of the weak and not to please ourselves; let each of us please our neighbor for the good, for building up" (Romans 15:1–2).

I recently experienced a powerful epiphany involving my daughter Shealagh. It came unexpectedly through a very ordinary occurrence. Shealagh reached up to scratch an itch on the back of her neck. At that moment I saw her in God's light. In witnessing this simple act, through no merit or effort of my own, I somehow came to a profound realization of how God sees us and loves us. This happened through the gift of a special grace. To God every moment of our lives, every act, save sin, no matter how insignificant, is special, beautiful, and endears us more so to Him. God's love is always pouring forth for us.

I received only a glimpse into this all-encompassing love of God for each of us. If I, the sinner that I am, can be moved to love by witnessing the innocence, specialness, fragility, beauty, simplicity, and dependency of my daughter when she merely scratched an itch, how much must God love us? It is incomprehensible.

Since we are created in God's image, and incorporated into Jesus, the second divine person of the Most Holy Trinity, and are temples of the Holy Spirit, since we are the beloved children of our Father, every act, even scratching one's neck, becomes divinized. "Your body, you know, is the temple of the Holy Spirit" (1 Corinthians 6:19, JB). What I was witnessing was Jesus, God and man, scratching His itch in the person of my daughter. We are capable of realizing this reality through the help of the Holy Spirit.

It is good to reflect on the fact that each of us was once a beloved, innocent five-year-old like my daughter Shealagh, no matter what has become of us in our lives, good or bad. That includes those who have committed the worse sins and atrocities. It also includes those people God has placed around us that we find difficult to love. Our Father never gives up on us. He always sees us as we were in our young age of innocence, and as we will become in the end, after the difficult, purifying, and magnificent paths of life. He is loving us unconditionally and arranging every moment and circumstance for our good, with the main goal that we spend all eternity perfectly happy with Him. This is the *main thing*!

We are called to love everyone—no exceptions. No exceptions? Yes, absolutely none! It is usually (though not always) easy for me to love my daughter Shealagh, but I am called to meet the daunting challenge of loving everyone, and accepting that others are not perfect, nor am I. "Treat others as you would like them to treat you. If you love those who love you, what thanks can you expect?" (Luke 6:31–33, JB).

When bearing a heavy cross like cancer, we are healed by God to hopefully have a greater capacity to be a little more tolerant and loving of others, to be more like our Lord Jesus who is utterly merciful. His mercy is available for everyone, and so we should make no exceptions with others. I, for one, recognize how far I fall short of being virtuous on a consistent basis, how impatient I can be with others, and how needy I am of God's mercy. I have been shown such incredible mercy. How can I withhold my mercy toward others?

With cancer God gives us a healing kick-start to begin to accept others no matter where they are in their life's journey. We have not walked in their shoes. We tend to be blind to our own shortcomings, but we can sure zero in on the faults of another from a mile away, and be ready to proclaim them from the rooftops. We all have a fallen human nature that is manifested in various ways. Not one of us is perfect. We are all a cross to our neighbor to some measure, indeed myself included.

Yes, we must love even our enemies: "love your enemies and do good" (Luke 6:35, JB). On a purely human level this is impossible, but with God's ever-ready help, it can be done. It must be done. "For God everything is possible" (Matthew 19:26, JB). And when we fail we must pick ourselves up, shake off the dust, and try to love again. I, for one, have had to shake off a mountain of dust over my lifetime, and the mountain is becoming Mount Everest.

During the course of my illness my family, friends, and even people I did not know personally have been tremendously supportive to me. I am truly awestruck and grateful for all of their help and prayers, which have been far reaching. But there have been times when I expected more from others than they had the capacity to deliver. I felt like they did not understand my cross completely. I seemed to expect an unattainable, infinite empathy and attention from them. But I need to remember that they are not God. Only God is God. The truth is that no one will understand and empathize with us to the degree that God does. No one will understand and empathize with me completely. Only God has the capacity to do so.

So we should not unduly place impossible expectations on others, including friends and relatives. We should be grateful for the help and understanding they are able to generously offer; each word, act, and prayer they offer is supremely valuable.

It is true that some individuals are able to console us more than others. They have a heightened understanding and empathy for us. These can often be family members who have journeyed with us through cancer or some other adversity, suffering with us every step of the way, or those we know or meet who have gone through a similar illness or cross. Because, like fellow soldiers who have fought and suffered side by side through the horror of battle can identify with each other like no other, so do we empathize with others in the same battle as us on a deeper level. Only those who have been through what you have been and are going through can truly understand the cross you and your family are carrying. But even those loved ones and fellow soldiers will be dim in their understanding compared to God, as only He has the capacity to know and empathize with us completely.

There is only One who knows and understands us more than we know and understand ourselves. He is the One who thoroughly identifies with each of us, the One who suffered and died on the cross for us, taking on all of our sins and infirmities. "And yet ours were the sufferings he bore, ours the sorrows he carried" (Isaiah 53:4, JB). He is the One who we are truly and completely one with. He is the only One who can give us absolute peace. He is the Lord Jesus. May we be grateful for the support and consolation of others which is so necessary and helpful, but may we look only to Jesus for complete healing and peace. "Only Jesus"! (Matthew 17:8, JB).

HEALING FROM OPPRESSION AND FEAR

"In love there can be no fear, but fear is driven out by perfect love: because to fear is to expect punishment, and anyone who is afraid is still imperfect in love" (1 John 4:18, JB).

September 24, 2011: Last night I had an experience or dream (only God knows which for sure) in which the devil was present, and I told him with assurance that any evil he does will only result in the end in giving greater glory to God, as God brings a tremendous good out of everything in His perfect providence, even evil. This incensed the devil so that he attacked me, but I knew that my soul was safe in Christ Jesus. Kathleen mentioned this morning when I shared this with her that she heard me groaning in my sleep last night.

Why am I sometimes afraid and anxious when things in general don't go according to my plan? Please, Lord Jesus, bless me with perfect love. I cannot achieve this on my own. Perhaps this is something that will always ebb and flow according to our weak human condition this side of heaven.

There are times, merely by the grace of God, that I seem to be entirely immersed in perfect love, when I am not at all afraid. I am invincible in Christ. Then there are times when my love is far from perfect. As a matter of fact, it seems to have dissipated all together. But I always know where to turn for strength. I merely need to turn to the One who strengthens me in my weakness. "So I shall be very happy to make my weaknesses my special boast so that the power of Christ may stay over me" (2 Corinthians 12:9–10, JB). And that power does stay over me at all times whether I feel it or not, because Jesus is "Faithful and True" (Revelation 19:2, JB). "For it is when I am weak that I am strong" (2 Corinthians 12:10, JB).

I have been highly blessed with a spring and summer 2011 of feeling fairly well and having lots of physical activity and time spent with my family, including playing light basketball, riding bikes, taking walks, playing board games, and watching good movies together. Life is a joy, especially when shared with beloved family members.

In July I underwent an advanced blood test that showed there is still CLL (Chronic Lymphocytic Leukemia) present in the blood. I also had a bone-marrow biopsy, which I think was at least my sixth since diagnosis. It makes a trip to the dentist a walk in the park. To put it in the simple terms my stem-cell doctor used to explain it me, there is still about 10 percent CLL including the aggressive 17p deletion cells in my bone marrow, but this is 75 percent less cancer than just before the stem-cell transplant. My good doctor is very encouraging that the donor cells will continue to attack the remaining cancer (graft versus leukemia) over the next six months and beyond, and eradicate it. There are, of course, no guarantees, and all would have preferred to see the cancer completely gone already, but the journey is progressing in a positive direction.

In about mid-July I began to feel quite sick. I was weak, had a low-grade fever, chills, and a limited appetite. I lost over ten pounds in about three weeks. I was itchy all over, and my joints were very painful, especially my back, so much so that I was unable to sleep more than a few hours per night, leaving me severely sleep deprived.

My back pain was unrelenting and excruciating. Eventually I was prescribed narcotic painkillers (which I reluctantly took only at night) and sleeping pills, which helped me to get some sleep, but which made me very drowsy around the clock. I regressed to not being able to drive a car for this reason.

This went on for about a month. I was able to be at my daughter Tara's beautiful wedding Mass and reception on July 30. God gave me a special burst of energy so I was able to be active throughout the wedding day and evening, despite my pain and illness. I even danced with my wife and every one of my twelve daughters, which would be no small feat for even a healthy man.

I developed a painful rash in the form of burns on my hands and wrists, to the extent they eventually peeled significantly. I then developed a rash on my upper torso. It turned out that all or most of the above symptoms (the back remaining in question) were a result of graft-versus-host disease (GVHD), wherein the donor stem cells graft and attack my body as foreign. It is actually a blessing in disguise to have some graft-versus-host disease, as this means the donor cells are active and are also attacking the cancer. Medications are provided to keep a proper balance so the graft versus leukemia (GVL) remains active without letting too much damage be done by the graft-versus-host disease.

In early/mid-August, my doctor put me on a fairly high dose (I had been on a low dose) of prednisone, a type of steroid, to control the GVHD. This worked wonders immediately in reducing my joint and back pain by about 90 percent, allowing me to go off the pain killers and sleeping pills, and to sleep somewhat normally again. Unfortunately there are negative side effects to the prednisone, including some significant muscle weakness, but I push through it just fine. The prednisone seems to be an excellent tradeoff, as I am feeling very well again. My doctor is gradually reducing the dosage. My rash seems to be in the healing process. I have some significant neuropathy (nerve damage from chemotherapy) in my lower legs, feet, and torso, but I don't let it stop me from being active. I just need to be careful with my movements because of the numbness, especially in my feet.

So, I have experienced yet another set of ups and downs along this long road of cancer. I must admit that I had been feeling so bad that I wondered if I would ever feel better again, and whether the end of my life was fast approaching. Then in a matter of a day or two with a medication adjustment I was feeling quite well again. This is yet another proof that God is ultimately in command of what happens to us, and when it happens. Certainly when one is feeling exceedingly ill and exhausted it is easy to fall into the oppression of fear and discouragement. But the truth does not change—God is arranging everything for the best. There is no reason to fear. We need only trust in Him. It takes a greater effort to trust in Jesus when things are at their most difficult, but that is precisely when He is there to do the heavy lifting for us.

When Christ is our *All* we have no fear. Is Jesus Christ my All? If not yet, am I willing to make Him my All, to let Him be my All?

"That evening they brought him many who were possessed by devils. He cast out the spirits with a word and cured all who were sick. This was to fulfill the prophecy of Isaiah: He took our sicknesses away and carried our diseases for us" (Matthew 8:16–17, JB).

Yes, devils exist, and they are quite active in stirring things up, trying to destroy our happiness, unity, and peace, doing all in their power to divert each of us from turning to Jesus with confidence for everything good. Jesus made it unequivocally clear that the devil is not only a liar, but *the father of lies.* "He was a murderer from the start; he was never grounded in the truth; there is no truth in him at all: when he lies he is drawing on his own store. because he is a liar, and the father of lies" (John 8:44, JB). So we should pay no attention whatsoever to what this enemy says or tries to instigate. When we fail to turn to Jesus the demons can easily wrap us around their devious fingers with their intelligence far superior to ours, and vent their unfathomable hate and rage against us. But we can be assured that they are powerless against Jesus. And when we turn to Jesus for protection and help we have no worries. With only a word He casts out devils—in fact, with no more than His willing it, it is done.

Jesus not only helps us by casting out devils, but He takes our sicknesses away, and He carries them for us. He took them to the cross. He takes them onto Himself, because there is a great deal more love in this vicarious suffering than if He had only cast away our diseases from a distance.

There are many types of diseases we need to be cured of, more than just the physical kind. The devils work against our weaknesses to try to instill fear, disunity, suspicion, impurity, and attacks against the dignity of the human person in diverse ways, including trying to warp the gift of our sexuality. The demonic tempts us to make a god of things, power, prestige, sex, ourselves. They attempt to delude us with the lie of moral relativism, attempting to convince us that we ourselves are the determiners of objective truth if there is any such thing, that we are the determiners of right and wrong, and that there is no such thing as sin—so that we think and live in a self-centered way as if we ourselves are gods.

The evil enemy likes to remain hidden where he can work more effectively through stealth. When he comes out in the open in his attacks against us it is a sign that he is frustrated and that we are not in his grips, that we are advancing the Kingdom of Jesus the Lord. Then we merely turn with complete confidence to Jesus who protects us most assuredly, though He may permit us to carry this cross a bit for a great good.

There is no need to fear or be oppressed by the devil, as long as we turn to Jesus for His always ready help. Bottom line, we are called to build our lives and eternity on the *impregnable Rock* of Jesus Christ. Jesus is the only true safe harbor, the only true complete fulfillment, the only true peace. Though everything God has made is good, all the things of this world will pass. We

227

should use everything God has given us for His glory. We enslave ourselves when we are fearful of losing anything outside of God. And that slavery is oppressive and cruel, a betrayer; it will never make us happy.

> I will show you what someone is like who comes to me, listens to my words, and acts on them. That one is like a person building a house, who dug deeply and laid the foundation on rock; when the flood came, the river burst against that house but could not shake it because it had been well built. But the one who listens and does not act is like a person who built a house on the ground without a foundation. When the river burst against it, it collapsed at once and was completely destroyed.

> Luke 6:47–49

In life, adversities can sometimes seem to come in a veritable overwhelming flood. But when we build our life and eternity on Jesus the Rock, nothing, and I mean nothing, can shake us.

"It was I who relieved your shoulder of the burden, your hands could drop the labourer's basket; you called in your trouble, so I rescued you. Hidden in the storm, I answered you, I tested you at the waters of Meribah" (Psalm 81: 6–7, JB). We are called to let go, not to try to control every outcome in our lives. We need to rest where true rest is found—that is, in Jesus. Jesus is our only true security. There is nothing to worry about. It may seem at times that He is hidden while we are in the midst of a storm, but we can be confident that He is there fully focused on us, seeing to the best for us. When we call out, His arms are always open to rescue us. He heals us by taking up our burden if we only allow Him.

HEALING THROUGH THE BREATH OF PRAYER

"There is need of only one thing. Mary has chosen the better part and it will not be taken from her" (Luke 10:42).

September 14, 2010: Today is the Feast day in the Catholic Church of the Triumph of the Cross. I have noticed for years how creation, and especially the sunrise and sunset, are generally, if not always, in sync with the liturgy of the Catholic Church. "You heavens, bless the Lord,/ praise and exalt him above all forever/....Sun and moon, bless the Lord;/ praise and exalt him above all forever" (Daniel 3:59,62).

This morning, as expected, I looked out the window during my morning prayer and was enthralled with the breathtaking sunrise, in which the entire horizon was blood red. Later in the morning as I drove to Mass with my family, we saw a white cloud formation in the distinct form of the cross spanning a major part of the horizon. The clouds were very unusual: quite thin where they made up the vertical and horizontal appearance of the cross. Earlier in the morning during prayer, when reading about the Feast day, I read: "Constantine the Great, not yet a Christian, while battling with Maxentius for the throne of the Roman Empire, prayed to the God of the Christians to aid him in his struggle. In answer to his prayer, a luminous cross or monogram of Christ appeared in the heavens bearing an inscription: 'In this sign you will conquer.' In gratitude for victory under this banner, over Maxentius at the Milvian Bridge, on October 28th, 312, Constantine had the sign of Christianity placed on the Roman standards and on the shields of his soldiers."[57]

I have witnessed this sort of exclamation of creation giving glory to God innumerable times in recent years, since I began to accept spiritual eyes to see this sort of thing.

Here's another example gleaned from my diary:

June 23, 2010, St. Ethelreda: There were major storms tonight in Frankfort. Afterward there was a rainbow along with an amazing sunset with wisps of clouds and bright sunshine filtering through, making it look like the sky was on fire. The weather seems to always be in sync with the Liturgy of the Church. Tomorrow is the solemnity of the Birth of St. John the Baptist.

"On the eve of St. John's day 'St. John's fires' were lighted on the hills and mountains in many countries as they are still lighted in some places. 'Scarce had the last rays of the setting sun died away, when all the world over, immense columns of flame arose from every mountaintop, and in an instant every town and village and hamlet was lighted up'" (Dom. P.L.P. Gueranger).[58] This is exactly how the sky appeared this evening, as if ablaze with fire.

An edited excerpt from my diary on the following morning:

June 24, 2010, Birth of St. John the Baptist: This morning there was a colorful, magnificent sunrise, in line with the canticle from Luke 1:76–79: "And you, child, will be called prophet of the Most High,/ for you will go before the Lord to prepare his ways,/ to give his people knowledge of salvation/ through the forgiveness of their sins,/ because of the tender mercy of our God/ by which the daybreak from on high will visit us/ to shine on those who sit in darkness and death's shadow,/ to guide our feet into the path of peace."

I also opened at random in my morning meditation to Isaiah 9:1: "The people who walked in darkness/ have seen a great light;/ Upon those who dwelt in the land of gloom a light has shown."

Yes, how can creation neglect to give glory to God?

For creation awaits with eager expectation the revelation of the children of God; for creation was made subject to futility, not of its own accord but because of the one who subjected it, in hope that creation itself would be set free from slavery to corruption and share in the glorious freedom of the children of God. We know that all creation is groaning in labor pains even until now; and not only that, but we ourselves, who have the firstfruits of the Spirit, we also groan within ourselves as we wait for adoption, the redemption of our bodies. For in hope we were saved.

Romans 8:19–24

There are signs of God's love, existence, and care all around us if only we open ourselves to the Holy Spirit's help to see things with supernatural eyesight. If only we had eyes to see. God will heal our inner sight if we ask Him. We will have no doubts about God's existence and His infinite love and care for each of us.

Look at all the times in the gospel when Jesus healed the blind that they might see, like the man blind from birth. This is a figure of being spiritually blind from birth. This sounds very applicable to me, and perhaps to many of you. "One thing I do know is that I was blind and now I see" (John 9:25).

This spiritual healing is there for the asking, I assure you. How could such a request not be in line with God's most holy and perfect will?

> For everyone who asks, receives; and the one who seeks, finds; and to the one who knocks, the door will be opened. What father among you would hand his son a snake when he asks for a fish? Or hand him a scorpion when he asks for an egg? If you then, who are wicked, know how to give good gifts to your children, how much more will the Father in heaven give the holy Spirit to those who ask him?
>
> Luke 11:10–13

Yes, we are wicked, but that fact only all the more entitles us to the mercy and good gifts of such a loving Redeemer. Yes, we have available to us the first fruits of the Spirit through whom we can pray. "The Spirit too comes to the aid of our weakness; for we do not know how to pray as we ought, but the Spirit itself intercedes with inexpressible groanings. And the one who searches hearts knows what is the intention of the Spirit, because it intercedes for the holy ones according to God's will" (Romans 8:26–27). And when our hearts are lifted up to the Most High God in awe of His signs in nature, are we not praying in the Spirit?

Prayer shores up hope. I am always encouraged and given hope by God through the meager effort of my prayer. If I show up to pray, God does the rest. I open my Bible at random every morning to converse with my best friend and Lord. Recently I encountered notations in my Bible where I had previously read the following passage:

> So many signs and wonders were worked among the people at the hands of the apostles that the sick were even taken out into the streets and laid on beds and sleeping-mats in the hope that at least the shadow of Peter might fall across some of them as he went past. People even came crowding in from the towns round about Jerusalem, bringing with them their sick and those tormented by unclean spirits, and all of them were cured.[59]

Acts 5:13–16, JB

I find it encouraging that I had noted in my Bible that I had opened at random to this same passage on the noteworthy dates of October 19, 2010, the one-year anniversary of my diagnosis, which is the Memorial of the North American Martyrs whose shrine my family and I made a pilgrimage to in July 2010; January 25, 2011, the date of my admission to the hospital for a stem-cell transplant; and January 28, 2011, the actual date of the transplant. And this cure has already been granted to me at least in that I am still alive at the time of writing this. None of us have any guarantee of living on this earth beyond the present moment. Thank You, Jesus, for the precious gem of this present moment.

Life is such a beautiful and precious gift. God's blessings are all around us reflected in all of creation. We can especially see the Face of God in the human faces around us—for me, especially in my wife and children. What a sublime dignity God has given us: we are created in His very image and likeness. "Then God said: 'Let us make man in our image, after our likeness'" (Genesis 1:26).

Prayer should be the pure air we breathe at every moment. Without breathing there is no life.

We are made to be perfectly happy. We seek happiness. Only God can make us entirely happy. No other person can completely satisfy this profound, innate desire. Only God can fulfill this—no one and nothing else. This is evident even in small things. My wife and I enjoy coffee. We found amaretto-flavored coffee to be our favorite. So we had it every day for a few months. We then found that we did not care for it so often and switched to another flavor. In a sense, this is one of many of the proofs of the existence of God. We will find that we will get sick of anything here on earth if we have too much of it too often. We are made for God. Only He can satiate our needs and desires for perfect love and happiness.

Do you know what a joy it is to open up your Bible every morning, and experience the Word of God? Do you know what a love affair the Lord is aching to have with you each morning, each day? Do you know how He desires to lift your soul and spirit up to heaven?

But how can spouses leave their love affair limited to their sublime conversations? Do not the Bridegroom, Jesus, and the bride, members of His Mystical Bride, the Church, desire to consummate their love? That is why, my friends, we cannot help but consume our Lord, to eat Him alive, to be one with Him, for us to be in Him, and for Him to be one in us! That ecstasy of consummation, of oneness, only happens in those Churches united entirely with the Catholic Church, in the reception of Jesus—Body, Blood, Soul, and Divinity—in the Eucharist. It is the ultimate joy and fulfillment! This is heaven on Earth! Jesus tells us with certainty: "I am the bread of life" (John 6:48, JB). If you are not Catholic, do you know what you are missing? Run, run to the nearest Catholic Church, and become one with Her! Am I making an imposition on your freedom? No, I am appealing to your free will; I am sharing with you the greatest gift, the source and summit of the Christian life, Jesus in the Eucharist!

There is someone, the enemy, who wants to do everything he can to stop us from receiving Jesus, His supreme gift to us,

Himself in the Eucharist. Jesus is the ultimate gracious Host who has prepared a banquet for us, a banquet where He gives Himself as the feast, as real food that brings us to eternal life. Oh, the devil despises the Eucharist, because He knows the supreme good that is wrought in the Eucharist for souls.

I dictated the above couple of paragraphs as I did for some of this book. When my daughter Fiona tried to play the tape on the transcription machine, it would not play, though there was definitely nothing physically wrongly with the tape. I examined it. It played just fine in my recorder. It played fine on its blank side. It moved freely on rewind and forward. Other tapes worked fine in the transcriber. I tested it in every way. It simply would not play in the transcriber. We eventually went through the more challenging means of transcription by playing it back with the hand recorder.

This is one of numerous examples I could share, many extremely awful to endure, of how the enemy of our souls, the evil one, attacks and tries to stop the work of the love of Jesus. When something like this happens, I rejoice, as it is an unmistakable sign that the work is going to have a very fruitful effect on a soul or souls. I am confident in the truth that Jesus, who is Love, is all powerful and will crush all the efforts of the enemy. This Jesus loved us so much that He became man and took on our sins and died for us. Jesus and every one of His members wins in the end. "Now since the children share in blood and flesh, he likewise shared in them, that through death he might destroy the one who has the power of death, that is, the devil, and free those who through fear of death had been subject to slavery all their life" (Hebrews 2:14–15).

What is Christ in the Eucharist? He is Love, Love, Love! He invites us to be one with Love. What did it cost Jesus to give us the Eucharist? Every drop of blood and water in His Body which poured out from His wounds on the cross. The water and blood from His side, in a sense, are the spiritual seminal fluid which consummates the marriage of Jesus the Bridegroom with His Church—with you, and me.[60] This is love. This is the Bridegroom laying down His life for his bride, the Church, to give His bride the very sustenance of His Body and Blood in the perpetual sacrifice, the Eucharist.

One of Jesus's last words on the cross was "I thirst" (John 19:28). For what does He thirst? He thirsts for you! He thirsts for me. He thirsts for souls. His love is a deep, unquenchable thirst. Do we only come to prayer to request favors or to refresh ourselves? Jesus longs, He thirsts to be consoled by our company, by our prayer. One does not need the perfect words, nor is it even required to speak in order to console a spouse or a close friend. One's presence is what is most important.

May we come always to Jesus in the *breath of prayer* and receive the healing He has in store for us in a thousand unanticipated, magnificent ways.

HEALING THROUGH A NEW LANGUAGE

"Be still and confess that I am God!" (Psalm 46:11).

When we are seriously ill we are healed in that we are prepared for a new, higher language. Jesus wishes to teach each of you this completely new language. In one minute flat you will be fluent. You will only need to practice it daily and to ask for God's help to perfect it.

As a matter of fact, I need only mention the name of this new language and you will immediately recognize it and become fluent. It is the language that Jesus Himself most often speaks. It is the most profound, brilliant, humble, and deep language of all time. It only takes a little effort and discipline to speak and understand it. It is the most intimate language. Nothing else compares. It cannot be written or spoken.

It is practical to live out this language almost anywhere, but it is best practiced before Jesus in the Blessed Sacrament. There it gives and receives its fullest expression.

It is the kind of language that only close friends can speak to each other. It cannot be spoken to a stranger. It emanates from the deepest part of the soul. It is not spoken with the mouth. It is not heard by the ears; yet one word can express everything. It is the very language that Jesus is speaking to you now. Can you hear Him?

Do you want to know this language? It is called *silence*. It is the language of total self-giving; it is the language of love.

Jesus implores us: "You must come away to some lonely place all by yourselves and rest for a while" (Mark 6:31, JB). He also says:

> But the Advocate, the Holy Spirit, whom the Father will send in my name, will teach you everything and remind you of all I have said to you. Peace I bequeath to you, my own peace I give you, a peace the world cannot give, this is my gift to you. Do not let your hearts be troubled or afraid.
>
> John 14:26–27, JB

The deep language of silence consists in presence to the other. What is most paramount in presence is not verbally spoken words but empathetically and lovingly accompanying the other. In keeping presence with God we are touched by Him. In keeping presence with another person we touch him or her, and we are touched in return, though there is nothing essentially physical about this touch. There is a oneness.

Have you ever experienced how consoling is the empathetic touch of another, particularly when we are suffering in some way? We may not physically feel the touch of God, but we experience it nonetheless in a much more profound manner in the superior part of our soul. Notice how only the closest family members and friends are comfortable in keeping silence with one another. When we are not secure in the other we feel compelled to speak as we tend to become very uncomfortable with silence. However, with those we are closest to, we are comfortable, content, and at peace in silence. Especially when we spend time in the real presence of Jesus in the Eucharist in silence, we are touched by Him, and we might say we touch and console Him, even become one with Him.

May we take advantage of the healing Jesus wants to shower upon us in spending some time with Him each day in the language of silence. He will listen to us, and we will learn to listen to Him; we will be healed in a thousand ways.

HEALING BY THE BREAD OF LIFE

"Then he took some bread, and when he had given thanks, broke it and gave it to them, saying, 'This is my body which will be given for you; do this as a memorial of me.' He did the same with the cup after supper, and said, 'This cup is the new covenant in my blood which will be poured out for you'" (Luke 22:19–20, JB).

Jesus heals more profoundly through the Eucharist than in any other way. He gives His Body and pours out His very life Blood for us. This was done once and for all in time, but the sacrifice is re-presented at every Mass.

According to the *Catechism of the Catholic Church*:

> In the New Testament, the memorial takes on new meaning. When the Church celebrates the Eucharist, she commemorates Christ's Passover, and it is made present the sacrifice Christ offered once for all on the cross remains ever present.[61] "As often as the sacrifice of the Cross by which 'Christ our Pasch has been sacrificed' is celebrated on the altar, the work of our redemption is carried out"[62] (CCC 1364).
>
> Because it is the memorial of Christ's Passover, the Eucharist is also a sacrifice. The sacrificial character of the Eucharist is manifested in the very words of institution:

"This is my body which is given for you" and "This cup which is poured out for you is the New Covenant in my blood."[63] In the Eucharist Christ gives us the very body which he gave up for us on the cross, the very blood which he "poured out for many for the forgiveness of sins" [64] (CCC 1365).

The Eucharist is thus a sacrifice because it *re-presents* (makes present) the sacrifice of the cross, because it is its *memorial* and because it *applies* its fruit:

"[Christ], our Lord and God, was once and for all to offer himself to God the Father by his death on the altar of the cross, to accomplish there an everlasting redemption. But because his priesthood was not to end with his death, at the Last Supper 'on the night when he was betrayed,' [he wanted] to leave to his beloved spouse the Church a visible sacrifice (as the nature of man demands) by which the bloody sacrifice which he was to accomplish once for all on the cross would be re-presented, its memory perpetuated until the end of the world, and its salutary power be applied to the forgiveness of the sins we daily commit." [65] CCC 1The sacrifice of Christ and the sacrifice of the Eucharist are *one single sacrifice*: "The victim is one and the same: the same now offers through the ministry of priests, who then offered himself on the cross; only the manner of offering is different." "And since in this divine sacrifice which is celebrated in the Mass, the same Christ who offered himself once in a bloody manner on the altar of the cross is contained and is offered in an unbloody manner... this sacrifice is truly propitiatory." [66]

CCC 1367

In the Eucharist that we see, we encounter Jesus with the eyes of faith, and we as Catholics are able to truly receive Him in Holy

Communion, Body, Blood, Soul, and Divinity, into our very body, soul, mind, and spirit. We become one with Him and He becomes one with us in the most sublime and real way. We become one with the Most Holy Trinity. It is most especially in the Eucharist that we encounter the love, mercy, and healing of Jesus.

Many say that the Eucharist is a symbol, Oh, no! The Eucharist is truly, really, substantially Jesus's Body and Blood, as taught for two thousand years by the Church and as prefigured for thousands of years as revealed in the Old Testament. What does Jesus have to say about this question? "I am the living bread which has come down from heaven. Anyone who eats this bread will live for ever; and the bread that I shall give is my flesh, for the life of the world" (John 6:51, JB). Also, "I tell you most solemnly, if you do not eat the flesh of the Son of Man and drink his blood, you will not have life in you. Anyone who does eat my flesh and drink my blood has eternal life, and I shall raise him up on the last day" (John 6:53–54, JB).

And, "whoever eats me will draw life from me" (John 6:57, JB). This is the *Ultimate Gift*, God Himself. This is as close as we can get to Jesus here on earth. The only difference in heaven will be that the veil will be lifted and He will no longer be hidden from our senses. We will see Him face-to-Face. "Jesus said to him, 'Have you come to believe because you have seen me? Blessed are those who have not seen and have believed'" (John 20:29).

Do you take the word of Jesus literally? Could the Truth, God and man, the wellspring of all virtue, who is incapable of lying, not be telling us the truth? He assures us that He is the truth. Jesus said to him, "I am the way and the truth and the life" (John 14:6). Well, many of Jesus's disciples were unwilling to accept and live Jesus's teaching on the Eucharist. Immediately after His discourse on the Eucharist, found in its entirety in the gospel of John, chapter 6, many of His disciples left Him. "After this, many of his disciples left him and stopped going with him" (John 6:66, JB). Though I am not a numerologist, this is an interesting number for the above scripture verse, 666. "Wisdom is needed here; one who understands can calculate the number of the beast, for it is a number that stands for a person. His number is six hundred and sixty-six" (Revelation 13:18).

Why did many of His disciples leave? Because they took Jesus literally that they were being invited to eat the flesh of the Son of Man and drink his blood! They were opposed to the teachings of Jesus regarding the Eucharist. They chose to leave Him. What a travesty of a choice! When we leave God, we leave everything. Jesus offers His very Self to us at the cost of His passion and death on the cross, and some choose to leave Him. Jesus, may we always stay close to You in good times and in seemingly bad. Jesus, please never permit me to leave You. Please have mercy on those who choose to keep You at a distance.

Not only do we get close to Jesus in the Eucharist, but we become one with Him, transformed into Him, divinized by Him, given eternal life by Him. This is the same Jesus we experience in the joy of receiving Him in Holy Communion, the same Jesus who walked the earth two thousand years ago, the same Jesus who suffered and died on the cross for us, the same Jesus who rose from the dead and ascended into heaven and is now seated at the right hand of the Father. Yes, Jesus is hidden from the senses. What we see, taste, feel, and smell seems to the senses to be bread and wine, but through the words of consecration by the priest in the Holy Mass these outward appearances have been truly and substantially changed into the Body, Blood, Soul, and Divinity of Jesus, the second person of the Holy Trinity. There is no longer bread and wine, only Jesus. And since there are three persons but one God, the Father and the Holy Spirit are also present in the Eucharist, loving us, sanctifying us. This supreme gift needs to be shared with others, inviting others to this transcendent banquet, where Jesus gives Himself to us totally. How can there not be lines daily in front of every Catholic Church with souls fervent to partake of this ultimate union with Christ Jesus?

The Eucharist is "the source and summit of the Christian life."[67] "The other sacraments, and indeed all ecclesiastical ministries and works of the apostolate, are bound up with the Eucharist and are oriented toward it. For in the blessed Eucharist is contained the whole spiritual good of the Church, namely Christ himself, our Pasch."[68]

CCC 1324

Yes, Jesus is the *source and summit*. All good comes from Jesus. Thus all good comes from Him in the Eucharist, because the Eucharist is Jesus! The good that flows from the Eucharist is ultimately meant to bring us to the Eucharist, in other words to Jesus, now and for all eternity.

What a beautiful and profound thing it is for each of us to be one flesh with our Divine Spouse, the Bridegroom here on earth, in the reality of Jesus giving Himself, His true Body, Blood, Soul, and Divinity, to us in Holy Communion. He is the Bridegroom, and we, the members of His Church, are His bride.

How often in Scripture is Jesus described as the bridegroom! Here are three examples:

Jesus answered them, "Can the wedding guests fast while the bridegroom is with them? As long as they have the bridegroom with them they cannot fast. But the days will come when the bridegroom is taken away from them, and then they will fast on that day" (Mark 2:19–20).

For he who has become your husband is your Maker;/ his name is the LORD of hosts;/ Your redeemer is the Holy One of Israel,/ called God of all the earth (Isaiah 54:5).

Let us rejoice and be glad/ and give him glory./ For the wedding day of the Lamb has come,/ his bride has made herself ready./ She was allowed to wear/ a bright, clean linen garment./ (The linen represents the righteous deeds of the holy ones.) Then the angel said to me, "Write this: Blessed are those who have been called to the wedding feast of the Lamb." And he said to me, "These words are true; they come from God."

Revelation 19:7–9

This Jesus, the Bridegroom, Who gives Himself to us as the Bread of Life in the Eucharist is the fulfillment of all of our deepest desires to be loved and to love. He is the complete fulfillment of the Old Testament, which so often prophesies about Jesus, as in the following example:

Yet it was our infirmities that he bore,/ our sufferings that he endured,/ While we thought of him as stricken,/ as one smitten by God and afflicted./ But he was pierced for our offenses,/ crushed for our sins,/ Upon him was the chastisement that makes us whole,/ by his stripes we were healed./ We had all gone astray like sheep,/ each following his own way;/ But the LORD laid upon him/ the guilt of us all./ Though he was harshly treated, he submitted/ and opened not his mouth;/ Like a lamb led to the slaughter/ or a sheep before the shearers,/ he was silent and opened not his mouth./ Oppressed and condemned, he was taken away,/ and who would have thought any more of his destiny?/ When he was cut off from the land of the living,/ and smitten for the sin of his people,/ A grave was assigned him among the wicked/ and a burial place with evildoers,/ Though he had done no wrong nor spoken any falsehood./ [But the LORD was pleased/ to crush him in infirmity.]/

If he gives his life as an offering for sin,/ he shall see his descendants in a long life,/ and the will of the LORD shall be accomplished through him./ Because of his affliction/ he shall see the light in fullness of days;/ Through his suffering, my servant shall justify many,/ and their guilt he shall bear./ Therefore I will give him his portion among the great,/ and he shall divide the spoils with the mighty,/ Because he surrendered himself to death/ and was counted among the wicked;/ And he shall take away the sins of many,/ and win pardon for their offenses.

Isaiah 53:4–12

Reception of Holy Communion is the *ultimate medicine* to heal us completely, body, mind, soul, and spirit, according to the perfect will of our Merciful Father, who truly and always knows what is best for us and is at work with His loving providence to that end. Remember, where we end up in eternity is what counts the most and is what God is most concerned with, though He loves to see attentively to every detail of our beautiful lives and to what we need here on earth as well.

So do not worry and say, "What are we to eat?" or "What are we to drink?" or "What are we to wear?" All these things the pagans seek. Your heavenly Father knows that you need them all. But seek first the kingdom [of God] and his righteousness, and all these things will be given you besides.

Matthew 6:31–33

In the Eucharist, Jesus pours out every drop of His love, His very self, into our souls. He actually does much more than heal us. He makes us infinitely better that we ever were, and ever could be without Him. He divinizes us! He transforms us into Himself, through no merit of our own, just as a patient often does nothing to heal himself but simply benefits from the medicine and/or treatment received, and the body's God-given capacity to heal.

I would like to go on to say much more about our Eucharistic Jesus, but it would take another entire book to merely scratch the surface. Besides, the reader will benefit much more through experience than by reading my words. If you are Catholic, I implore you to participate in the Mass and receive Jesus daily. There is nothing greater you can do with the precious gift of your time. Nothing! Whether Catholic or not, visit Jesus in the tabernacle or an adoration chapel. Kneel or sit in His presence, and He will win you, heal you in a thousand ways, and heap more gifts upon you than you could ever imagine. Most especially He will give you His peace and mercy.

It is all a gift! Praise the Lord!

HEALING THROUGH DEATH

"Amen, amen, I say to you, you will weep and mourn, while the world rejoices; you will grieve, but your grief will become joy. When a woman is in labor, she is in anguish because her hour has arrived; but when she has given birth to a child, she no longer remembers the pain because of her joy that a child has been born into the world. So you also are now in anguish. But I will see you again, and your hearts will rejoice, and no one will take your joy away from you" (John 16:20–22).

Death is the definitive event we must all pass through. For those of us who have sincerely repented, sought the mercy of God, and are in a state of grace, death is a birth into eternal life with God, His angels, and all those who are saved by the Blood of the Lamb. "They have washed their robes white again in the blood of the Lamb" (Revelation 7:14, JB).

In death we are actually born into eternal life. To borrow and expound upon an analogy from the Venerable Archbishop Fulton J. Sheen, a baby in the womb might tell himself that it is quite comfortable in there, and that he would prefer to stay there as the world outside that birth canal is mysterious, scary, and unknown. But eventually out he comes, born into life outside the womb, like it or not—and what a beautiful gift life is! Well, our birth into eternal life may seem scary, and we try to put it off as long as we can, but it will be immensely superior to being born of our mothers, as long as we choose to do our best to live and love, and to turn to Jesus for mercy and forgiveness for our failings.[69] Jesus loves to pour His mercy out on us. Why else would He have died on the cross for us?

We may have a stopover in purgatory to complete our purification before entering the presence of our King, Jesus, but we will eventually find ourselves enjoying the beatific vision, experiencing our Lord Jesus face-to-Face eternally. We want to be our very best before we come into His majestic presence, because we love and respect Him. "That day will begin with fire, and the fire will test the quality of each man's work. If his structure stands up to it, he will get his wages; if it is burnt down, he will be the loser, and though he is saved himself, it will be as one who has gone through fire" (1 Corinthians 3:13–15, JB).

After all, deep and truly authentic love this side of heaven is always mixed with pain and sorrow.[70] This is a condition of becoming one with Perfect Love, Jesus, and which is associated with the cross that leads to the resurrection and perfect happiness for all eternity. This pain and sorrow is the seed of divine, painless, blissful, eternal love, where we are face-to-Face with our beloved Jesus. "Let your face smile on your servant, save me in your love" (Psalm 31:16, JB). The fruit of the cross is no less than our very divinization.

Purgatory is a merciful but painful place and process of purification. Only pain is really effective in purifying us. We are all in need of purification. But the mixed bag of good news is that I believe those of us whom God has permitted to carry heavy crosses like cancer will have completed much, if not all, of our purgatory here on earth. The best news is that those of us who land in purgatory are certain to have heaven as our next destination. That is the only place we can possibly go from there. Even if we are there longer than we might prefer, it will be a very short stay compared to eternity in heaven.

When we are at peace with God it is easier, with His help, to abandon and surrender ourselves to the mystery of death when it comes. But in the meantime we should not measure our life by its future length, but by the life we have been gifted with today. Every moment is a gem. We can make that gem shine by the way we live our lives, with God's essential assistance.

> But now Christ has been raised from the dead, the firstfruits of those who have fallen asleep. For since death came through a human being, the resurrection of the dead came also through a human being. For just as in Adam all die, so too in Christ shall all be brought to life, but each one in proper order: Christ the firstfruits; then, at his coming, those who belong to Christ; then comes the end, when he hands over the kingdom to his God and Father, when he has destroyed every sovereignty and every authority and power. For he must reign until he has put all his enemies under his feet. The last enemy to be destroyed is death, for "he subjected everything under his feet." But when it says that everything has been subjected, it is clear that it excludes the one who subjected everything to him. When everything is subjected to him, then the Son himself will [also] be subjected to the one who subjected everything to him, so that God may be all in all.

1 Corinthians 15:20–28

Yes, Jesus puts death to the sword that we may live with Him forever, that God may be all in all. Jesus, You are my All!

> Jesus answered them, "The hour has come for the Son of Man to be glorified. Amen, amen, I say to you, unless a grain of wheat falls to the ground and dies, it remains just a grain of wheat; but if it dies, it produces much fruit.

Whoever loves his life loses it, and whoever hates his life in this world will preserve it for eternal life. Whoever serves me must follow me, and where I am, there also will my servant be. The Father will honor whoever serves me."

John 12:23–26

Isn't this an amazing example that Jesus left for us to do our best to emulate? He identified His death on the cross as His *glorification*, not because His pain and agony was good in itself, but because of the infinite good that would come of it. We are all grains that must die to bear the ultimate fruit. Jesus went before us. We, His servants, must follow; and we will be honored by the Father.

It is good to remember that we are called to die to ourselves while we live here on earth, to work on not being self-centered but God-centered and other-centered, to truly love our neighbors and, yes, our enemies. This way we will preserve our life for eternal life. We need to put the things of this world in proper perspective, using them for their good purpose, but not being so attached that we put them before God. We can accomplish all this with God's help.

In facing our mortality, whether sick or healthy, it might be good to reflect on the fact that in one hundred and twenty years or less, truly a short time, not a single person living on this earth out of billions will still be alive. We are all mortal beings. Each of us is building his eternity with the choices we make in our lives. We will all exit this life, being born into eternity, and face the judgment of our all-powerful yet merciful God and savior, Jesus Christ. If only we could keep this inescapable fact in mind in an encouraging, not oppressing, way. Life is truly short and fleeting for the strongest and healthiest of us. We should see each day as a gift, a unique gem, as an opportunity to grow in our love for God and neighbor through our prayers, actions, and words. God, please help me to take my own advice!

But the souls of the just are in the hand of God,/ and no torment shall touch them./ They seemed, in the view of the foolish, to be dead;/ and their passing away was thought an affliction/ and their going forth from us, utter destruction./ But they are in peace.

Wisdom 3:1–3

It is profound to contemplate the mystery of the awesome things in store for the just. Uh oh! Who is just? None of us are! What are we to hope for? Our hope is fulfilled in Jesus! It is the Just One, Jesus, who justifies us, as long as we repent and seek His mercy. "These are the sort of people some of you were once, but now you have been washed clean, and sanctified, and justified through the name of the Lord Jesus Christ and thought the Spirit of our God" (1 Corinthians 6:11, JB). We will never be perfect here on earth, though we are called to try our best motivated by love. But never fear, Jesus justifies us nonetheless and pours forth His inexhaustible mercy upon us. We are all in need of His mercy. In Him we find peace.

If we can keep the thought with us that each of us will eventually die, sooner or later, currently healthy or not, I think that although we won't become perfect, we will live better, more virtuous lives with our priorities in better order—especially with regard to things like God, family, friends, and generous service to others. Keeping the reality of our eventual death here on earth opens the door for the Wisdom Whom God wishes to pour into our minds and souls. "Teach us to count how few days we have and so gain wisdom of heart" (Psalm 90:12, JB).

As beautiful as life is here on earth we are truly healed through death. Yes, at death we experience our final consequence for original sin. "For dust you are and to dust you shall return" (Genesis 3:19, JB). Death was not in God's original plan for us. He did not want our first parents, Adam and Eve, to sin, or to die, but once they sinned He brought an infinitely great good out of it. We return to the citation: "O truly necessary sin of Adam, destroyed completely by the Death of Christ! O happy fault that earned so great, so glorious a Redeemer!"[71]

God is in no way vindictive. I am convinced that He would not have permitted death as a consequence of original sin, if He did not plan an infinitely great good to arise out of it. That is not to say that death is not a hard cross. It is! But God assures us through His Word in Scripture that He is bringing something grand out of it for us: "We know that by turning everything to their good God co-operates with all those who love him, with all those that he has called according to his purpose" (Romans 8:28, JB). And again, by everything God means everything, not excluding death. "Amen, I say to you, today you will be with me in Paradise." (Luke 23:42–43)We truly have nothing to fear. Only Jesus can heal us from our natural fears. We are called to trust in Him. He will relieve our burden.

> Do not let your hearts be troubled. Trust in God still, and trust in me. There are many rooms in my Father's house; if there were not, I should have told you. I am going now to prepare a place for you, and after I have gone and prepared you a place, I shall return to take you with me; so that where I am you may be too.
>
> John 14:1–3, JB

Having said all this, it is good to strive to prolong our lives through reasonable means. Life is such a magnificent gift in so many ways. God wants us to live to the full and make the best of our lives especially for the good of others and His glory. Christ came to give us life and that we might have it more abundantly. "I have come so that they may have life and have it to the full" (John 10:10, JB).

Jesus brought the dead He encountered back to life. He, the giver of Life, knows very well its value. "This God of ours is a God who saves, to the Lord Yahweh belong the ways of escape from death" (Psalm 68:20, JB).

Jesus wept at the death of His friend Lazarus before raising him from the dead. His empathy and compassion are infinitely beyond all the empathy and compassion ever mustered by everyone combined who ever lived, and will ever live. "Jesus said in great distress, with a sigh that came straight from the heart, 'Where have you put him?' They said, 'Lord, come and see' Jesus wept; and the Jews said, 'See how much he loved him!'" (John 11:33–37, JB). And this is how much Jesus loves each of us, unconditionally and infinitely.

Jesus brought Lazarus back to life. "He cried in a loud voice, 'Lazarus, here! Come out!' The dead man came out, his feet and hands bound with bands of stuff and a cloth round his face. Jesus said to them, 'Unbind him, let him go free'" (John 11:43–44, JB). Only Jesus can unbind us, and set us free!

But we should keep in mind that we are on a transitory pilgrimage here on earth leading to eternal life in heaven. Everyone Jesus brought back to life eventually died. They were merely given more precious time on earth to complete their mission.

For each of us who have sincerely repented and sought His mercy, I think we can safely say that death, followed by a merciful, purifying period of time in purgatory for many of us and our entry into heaven, is the definitive healing God has in store for us. At that point all pain and suffering will be behind us. There will only be peace, happiness, and total fulfillment as we behold the Face of God.

I ask you, what can separate us from the inexhaustible love of God? Nothing!

> For I am convinced that neither death, nor life, nor angels,
> nor principalities, nor present things, nor future things, nor

powers, nor height, nor depth, nor any other creature will be able to separate us from the love of God in Christ Jesus our Lord.

Romans 8:38–39

Death cannot kill love. As a matter of fact, it inflames it. May we always remember and pray with deep love for our beloved family members and friends, as well as those with no one to remember or pray for them; for those who are in heaven and purgatory surely, with God's assistance, remember and watch over us. We pray with hope and confidence in the mercy of God that they are already in heaven, or on their way there through the mercy of purgatory.

When the time comes that our Lord calls us and tells us that our time is up we should be ready, with His help, to meet Him in peace, seeking and trusting with complete confidence in His mercy. We will, after all, be meeting the One we have loved and Who loves us.

And we have confident hope that we will hear our beloved Jesus welcome us with the words: "Well done, good and faithful servant" (Matthew 25:23, JB).

HEALING THROUGH REDEMPTION AND RESURRECTION

"I consider that the sufferings of this present time are as nothing compared with the glory to be revealed for us" (Romans 8:18).

I used to worry about many things, rush through things just to get them out of the way, so I could get on to the next best thing; but as it turned out the current thing always was and is the best thing, the real thing, the only thing. This beautiful life is a gift, a gem, no moment or circumstance excluded. We have to live it to the full, as this life is passing quickly for all of us on our way to the inescapable reality of death, judgment, and eternity.

Luke 7:11–15: "Soon afterward he journeyed to a city called Nain, and his disciples and a large crowd accompanied him. As he drew near to the gate of the city, a man who had died was being carried out, the only son of his mother, and she was a widow. A large crowd from the city was with her." There is much in common in this passage with Jesus and His mother, Mary, as well as with our own life and death. Jesus also was the only son of Mary, and she was a widow.

"When the Lord saw her, he was moved with pity for her and said to her, 'Do not weep.'" This widow was obviously weeping, since Jesus asked her not to. This is a figure of how the Blessed

Virgin Mary weeps when we are dead in sin, imploring the abundant mercy of her Son, Jesus, toward us. Jesus is always filled with intense pity and compassion for us. Can we even imagine how much He loves?

"He stepped forward and touched the coffin." It was Jesus who took the initiative and stepped forward. He always takes the initiative with us. Oh, what love, life, and power are in this touch of Jesus! Time, creation, and the very laws of nature stop enraptured in wonder at the healing balm contained in the delicate touch of Jesus! How can a beloved child of God remain dead in the Savior's presence?

"At this the bearers halted, and he said, 'Young man, I tell you, arise!' The dead man sat up and began to speak, and Jesus gave him to his mother." When we die physically our Mother, Mary, weeps for us. She intercedes with her tears which always move our Lord Jesus to answer her prayers in the affirmative. Her will is always in accord with the will of God. Upon our personal death we pray, hope, and believe we will hear the words of our Lord Jesus, who has all power over life and death: *I tell you, arise!* What beautiful consoling words these will be to hear. And the best part will be when He will give us to our Mother, Mary, to whom we owe more than we can comprehend.

Venerable Archbishop Fulton J. Sheen tells us that "no dead person ever stayed dead" in the presence of Jesus.[72] He will not abandon us. "I will not leave you orphans; I will come to you. In a little while the world will no longer see me, but you will see me, because I live and you will live. On that day you will realize that I am in my Father and you are in me and I in you" (John 14:18–20).

But some of you may protest that you have squandered your life, that you have lived in sin with little or no practice of religion or worship your entire life. Is it too late? No! It is never too late while we are still alive in this world. I can assure you that in God's justice, which is resplendent with mercy and generosity, "the last will be first, and the first will be last" (Matthew 20:16). This is not because I said it, but because Jesus, God and man, said it! Repent and seek God's mercy and you will move to the front of the line, receiving the same gift of eternal life in heaven as one who has borne the day's burden and the heat working hard to live a virtuous life and give glory to God during his whole life (I am not one of them). And you who have lived a virtuous holy life your entire life (if any such persons exist) are forbidden to be prideful or envious. Is our Lord Jesus not free to do what He wishes and be generous with His gifts? Of course, none of us goes to heaven based on our own merit, but only on the copious mercy of Jesus.

I hope the reader will take solace in the following passage:

> The kingdom of heaven is like a landowner who went out at dawn to hire laborers for his vineyard. After agreeing with them for the usual daily wage, he sent them into his vineyard. Going out about nine o'clock, he saw others standing idle in the marketplace, and he said to them, "You too go into my vineyard, and I will give you what is just." So they went off. [And] he went out again around noon, and around three o'clock, and did likewise. Going out about five o'clock, he found others standing around, and said to them, "Why do you stand here idle all day?" They answered, "Because no one has hired us." He said to them, "You too go into my vineyard." When it was evening the owner of the vineyard said to his foreman, "Summon the laborers and give them their pay, beginning with the last and ending with the first." When those who had started about five o'clock came, each received the usual daily wage. So when the first came, they thought that they would receive more, but each of them also got the usual wage. And on receiving it they grumbled against the landowner, saying, "These last ones worked only one hour, and you have made them equal to us, who bore the day's burden and the heat." He said to one of them in reply, "My friend, I am not cheating you.

259

Did you not agree with me for the usual daily wage? Take what is yours and go. What if I wish to give this last one the same as you? [Or] am I not free to do as I wish with my own money? Are you envious because I am generous?" Thus, the last will be first, and the first will be last.

Matthew 20:1–16

No matter what the time, season, and circumstance of our life, now is the time to get to work in the vineyard of our Lord Jesus. We see in this parable that it was the landowner that continually sought out the idle to put them to work in his vineyard. This is exactly how Jesus operates with us. He is always taking the initiative, seeking us out, and inviting us into His vineyard, which is the most luscious, stunning vineyard in the universe.

When invited into the vineyard of Jesus, go now! None of the workers in this parable put it off once invited. None waited to see if there would be another opportunity later. God is infinitely generous, but our lives and opportunities on earth are limited. We should never presume there will be another opportunity. What's more, why wait? The work in this vineyard is not difficult. It is sweet, and the wages are infinite.

May we be given the grace like St. Paul not to fear death.

My eager expectation and hope is that I shall not be put to shame in any way, but that with all boldness, now as always, Christ will be magnified in my body, whether by life or by death. For to me life is Christ, and death is gain.

Philippians 1:20–21

Death has been slaughtered. It is gone! Jesus put death to death by His own death and resurrection. "Where, O death, is your victory?/ Where, O death, is your sting?" (1 Corinthians 15:55).

Many of you may ask, "How are dead people raised, and what sort of body do they have when they come back?" (1 Corinthians 15:35–26, JB). Well, neither I nor the Church has all the answers. Some details are a mystery, which is fine, because God has revealed plenty to console us and give us hope. I share some of the official teachings of the Catholic Church from the *Catechism of the Catholic Church* regarding these questions for the reader's benefit. These revealed truths can be taken for certain.

> *What is "rising"?* In death, the separation of the soul from the body, the human body decays and the soul goes to meet God, while awaiting its reunion with its glorified body. God, in his almighty power, will definitively grant incorruptible life to our bodies by reuniting them with our souls, through the power of Jesus' Resurrection (CCC 997).
>
> *Who will rise?* All the dead will rise, "those who have done good, to the resurrection of life, and those who have done evil, to the resurrection of judgment"[73] (CCC 998).
>
> *How?* Christ is raised with his own body: "See my hands and my feet, that it is I myself";[74] but he did not return to an earthly life. So, in him, "all of them will rise again with their own bodies which they now bear," but Christ "will change our lowly body to be like his glorious body," into a "spiritual body":[75]
>
> "But someone will ask, 'How are the dead raised? With what kind of body do they come?' You foolish man! What you sow does not come to life unless it dies. And what you sow is not the body which is to be, but a bare kernel....What is sown is perishable, what is raised is imperishable....The dead will be raised imperishable....For this perishable nature must put on the imperishable, and this mortal nature must put on immortality[76]" (CCC 999).
>
> This "how" exceeds our imagination and understanding; it is accessible only to faith. Yet our participation in

261

the Eucharist already gives us a foretaste of Christ's transfiguration of our bodies:

"Just as bread that comes from the earth, after God's blessing has been invoked upon it, is no longer ordinary bread, but Eucharist, formed of two things, the one earthly and the other heavenly: so too our bodies, which partake of the Eucharist, are no longer corruptible, but possess the hope of resurrection"[77] (CCC 1000).

In expectation of that day, the believer's body and soul already participate in the dignity of belonging to Christ. This dignity entails the demand that he should treat with respect his own body, but also the body of every other person, especially the suffering:

"The body [is meant] for the Lord, and the Lord for the body. And God raised the Lord and will also raise us up by his power. Do you not know that your bodies are members of Christ?...You are not your own....So glorify God in your body"[78] (CCC 1004).

God did not send His Son to condemn us, but that we might be saved through Him. May we never doubt this!

"No one has gone up to heaven except the one who has come down from heaven, the Son of Man. And just as Moses lifted up the serpent in the desert, so must the Son of Man be lifted up, so that everyone who believes in him may have eternal life. For God so loved the world that he gave his only Son, so that everyone who believes in him might not perish but might have eternal life. For God did not send his Son into the world to condemn the world, but that the world might be saved through him."

John 3:13–1

So, count on the fact that there is the ultimate healing of a resurrection awaiting each of us. Christ will transfigure our bodies. They will be better than ever. For those who humble themselves and repent seeking the mercy of Jesus there is redemption and everlasting happiness and peace. Thank You, Jesus!

HEALING
THROUGH POURING

"The love of God has been poured into our hearts by the Holy Spirit, which has been given us" (Romans 5:6, JB).

We will be most happy when we become *pourers:* Matthew 19:16–22: "Now someone approached him [Jesus] and said, 'Teacher, what good must I do to gain eternal life?'" Note the question. The man is asking about what good he himself must do. He seems to be asking what the bare essentials are that he is required to do. This, unfortunately, is an example of *dripping* as opposed to *pouring.* "He answered him, 'Why do you ask me about the good? There is only One who is good.'" In other words we ourselves cannot muster any good. We are only able to be good or accomplish good through the One who is good, our Blessed Lord.

Jesus adds: "If you wish to enter into life, keep the commandments." Note that Jesus is answering the particular question posed by the man. He is providing him with the bare minimum the man must do to enter into life. This is tied into the law of the Old Testament. The commandments, every iota, are still valid.

> Do not think that I have come to abolish the law or the prophets. I have come not to abolish but to fulfill. Amen, I say to you, until heaven and earth pass away, not the smallest

letter or the smallest part of a letter will pass from the law, until all things have taken place. Therefore, whoever breaks one of the least of these commandments and teaches others to do so will be called least in the kingdom of heaven. But whoever obeys and teaches these commandments will be called greatest in the kingdom of heaven.

Matthew 5:17–19

However, Jesus proposes something much more profound. Returning to Matthew 19:16–22: "He asked him, 'Which ones?' And Jesus replied, 'You shall not kill; you shall not commit adultery; you shall not steal; you shall not bear false witness; honor your father and mother'; and 'you shall love your neighbor as yourself.'" Here our Blessed Lord repeats the bare-essential commandments, which the man was well aware of. The young man said to him, "All of these I have observed. What do I still lack?" Something was gnawing at the man's soul. He was not happy. He sensed that he was lacking something, that he was being invited in his soul, in his interior, to something deeper than a superficial, perhaps even self-centered, keeping of the commandments, of the law.

"Jesus said to him, 'If you wish to be perfect, go, sell what you have and give to [the] poor, and you will have treasure in heaven.'" Note that Jesus changes the premise here. He says, "If you wish to be perfect." The question is no longer about the bare-minimum pursuit of gaining one's salvation, of finding out what the minimum is that one must do to scarcely slip into heaven in the end. He says, "If you wish to be perfect." Now the object, the goal, being proposed is perfection. This is based on the supremely higher *law of love*. This calls for more than strict observance of the law. Jesus invites the young man as He invites us to surrender everything, to let go of everything we have made into little gods. "Go, sell what you have and give to [the] poor." He proposes that we make God *our All*. That we let go of every attachment that we have, and that we become *pourers*, that is *total givers*, being focused entirely on God's glory and on others.

Jesus says, "Then come, follow me." Jesus went first. He taught us what it means to be a pourer. He gave everything. Jesus, God, the second person of the Most Holy Trinity, became man so He could suffer and die on the cross, pour out every drop of His blood, and every drop of water in His Body, out of true and perfect love for us. "But one soldier thrust his lance into his side, and immediately blood and water flowed out" (John 19:34). If our Master gave everything, then we are called to do the same, and He will help us to accomplish this. We are not capable on our own. "There is only One who is good."

Returning to Matthew 19:16–22: "When the young man heard this statement, he went away sad, for he had many possessions." This poor young man—and we pray that he later came to a deeper conversion—went away sad, for he had many attachments. He placed many things before God. What are our attachments— money, health, power, things, prestige, sex, pleasure? Using the things that we truly need in this world is fine, but we cannot put them before God. God must be our All, because we are made for Him. We will only be happy when we allow Him to become Everything for us, to be our All. This is another example of how God's ways are not our ways.

The world tells us that the more successful we are, the more things and toys we have, the happier we will be. This is absolutely not true. Only God can fill our good and God-given desire for perfect happiness. God loves us so much that He often permits us to find Him the *hard way*, as it is the *only way* that can break through the walls we have built. He allows us to become miserable once we have satiated ourselves with the things of the world and found ourselves dejected and bilious. We can never seem to get enough of anything, because nothing but God fulfills our intrinsic desire for perfect happiness. Every one of us has been created to be entirely happy. It is right that we should pursue happiness. But only God can fill this ache and desire imprinted deep inside of each of us. We are right to want everything. But the things of this world are not it. He is!

We are called to be *pourers, not drips*. Pourers pour out all they have at every moment for God and others, not concerned with keeping anything for themselves. They do so quietly, trying not to draw undue attention to themselves. These are truly happy people.

"Jesus was at Bethany in the house of Simon the leper, when a woman came to him with an alabaster jar of the most expensive ointment, and poured it on his head as he was at table" (Matthew 26:6–8, JB). This woman did not make a spectacle of dripping out her treasure, but generously poured it out completely on Jesus.

Drips on the other hand tend to be self-centered, unhappy people who make an exhibition of the little they do manage to drip out, sometimes doing so mainly with the motive of gaining human respect, which really counts for nothing.

Even when we are in need we can still give something to others, be it a couple dollars, our physical help and presence when we are able, our encouraging words, or our efficacious prayers; and we can form an intention of offering all of our sufferings and joys to Jesus for the benefit of others.

> Then David said to his son Solomon, "Be strong, stand firm; be fearless, be dauntless and set to work because Yahweh God, my God, is with you. He will not fail you or forsake you before you have finished all the work to be done for the house of Yahweh."
>
> 1 Chronicles 28:20–21, JB

We see here how God is in command and is sustaining us until the moment, only He knows, when He will call us from this world. He will not fail us. This passage also encourages us to be pourers who exercise our particular talents in fulfilling whatever mission God has for us with the purpose of helping to bring souls to Christ and giving glory to God.

I have leukemia. Medically there is a significant chance that I will die from this, though I may live for a long time; I may even be healed. In a way this is irrelevant. What counts is what we do with the gift of our lives, what we do with the gift of each day, with each moment. Every one of us is dying. Every one of us is living at this moment. We are not guaranteed tomorrow; none of us are. We need to live our lives well, without fear.

So many of the great saints did their most important work when they were very ill, even with terminal diseases. St. Maximilian Kolbe was diagnosed with potentially terminal, advanced tuberculosis as a young man.[79] He lived on for decades, doing some of the greatest work the Church has ever seen. When his illness was at the worst, he was working all the harder, and God was bringing great fruit out of this work sated with the redemptive suffering of the cross.

When did Christ do His greatest work? On the cross, in His death, culminating in His resurrection, to redeem us all. We have a God who went before us, who took His own medicine as the great Venerable Archbishop Fulton J. Sheen has held.[80]

Another example is St. Pio who suffered serious illnesses much of his life, but nonetheless kept at his exhausting work as a priest and religious, day in and day out, including hearing confessions twelve hours per day.

What if St. Pio and St. Maximilian Kolbe had fearfully opted out of service, waiting around to die? My guess is that they may have very well died much sooner, or at best they would have lived on in mediocrity with much of the fruit of their lives lost. Sacrifice and service invigorated them. God sustained and blessed them for their heroic efforts.

Why do I, as the happily married father of nineteen children, fourteen living, have this really serious illness of leukemia? In some sense this is a mystery to me, but one thing is certain, it is permitted by God and is therefore part of His most perfect, holy will from which He brings out a tremendously greater good. "We know that all things work for good for those who love God, who are called according to his purpose" (Romans 8:28).

Perhaps one of the many reasons that God led you to read this book at this time is so you will be in some way consoled and encouraged to make the very best out of your life, whether sick or healthy. Many who are sick are going to outlive those who are seemingly healthy at this time. But how long I live is beside the point. What am I doing with my life? Am I huddling in a corner, afraid, waiting to see whether I will survive this current illness or cross; or am I courageously living my life and using my gifts for the glory of God and the good of others? Or are things going seemingly so well in my life that I have fooled myself into thinking that I do not need God? "So even those whom God allows to suffer must trust themselves to the constancy of the creator and go on doing good" (1 Peter 4:19, JB). There is no question that we are energized when we put our talents to work.

St. Maximilian Kolbe did not bury himself in a corner wondering if he was going to die from his illness. Rather he spent decades doing amazingly fruitful apostolic service and ended up dying, not of his illness, but of a total gift of himself in gallantly laying down his life for his fellow man as a martyr in Auschwitz concentration camp. The things that we fear more often than not never come to fruition. As a matter of fact, we cause ourselves much unnecessary agony in worrying about things that are really outside of our control. They are in the control of our most loving Heavenly Father. "Do not worry about tomorrow; tomorrow will take care of itself. Sufficient for a day is its own evil" (Matthew 6:34).

It is interesting how often the word *pour* is used in Scripture. An example is in Matthew 26:26–29 (JB). Here Jesus, God and man, our Lord and Savior, is the ultimate Pourer.

Now as they were eating, Jesus took some bread, and when he had said the blessing he broke it and gave it to the disciples. "Take it and eat;" he said "this is my body." Then he took a cup, and when he had returned thanks he gave it to them. "Drink all of you from this," he said "for this is my blood, the blood of the covenant, which is to be poured out for many for the forgiveness of sins."

This was the institution of the Eucharist. At every Mass the bread and wine are actually and truly changed into the Body and Blood of Jesus Christ.

Jesus taught us what it means to be a pourer. He suffered and died on the cross for each of us, because He loves us. His love is *agape* (a classical Greek word), the highest form of love that is totally unconditional and selfless. He literally poured out all the water and blood in His Body, when His side was pierced with a lance. "When they came to Jesus, they found he was already dead, and so instead of breaking his legs one of the soldiers pierced his side with a lance; and immediately there came out blood and water" (John 19:33–35, JB).

Yes, He poured out every drop of blood, because He who was sinless took on our sins (see 2 Corinthians 5:21), and "sin is in the blood."[81] In this way He saved, healed, and completely cleansed each of us who are willing to repent and accept His bountiful mercy.

The water represents the living waters of Baptism and the Holy Spirit. The blood represents the Most Holy Eucharist. Every time we as Catholics partake of Holy Communion we are being transformed more into Christ and given an increased capacity to be *pourers* like Jesus Himself. We are given supernatural graces to help us rise above our natural selfishness to be selfless servants of God and our neighbor.

Jesus is the *definitive pourer*. He pours forth the very third person of the Trinity, the Holy Spirit, God Himself, into our souls. "Exalted at the right hand of God, he received the promise of the holy Spirit from the Father and poured it forth, as you [both] see and hear" (Acts 2:33). We become temples of God! Particularly through partaking in the Eucharist we actually become divinized through no power of our own. Everything from God is a gift, because He is the perfect and constant *Giver*, the ultimate *Pourer*.

Those of us who have cancer or carry other heavy crosses often are healed in the sense of receiving a heightened understanding of our mission to be *pourers*. When we are selfish and self-centered, we tend not to be happy. When we serve others as Jesus did, giving all we can in whatever way we can, be it deeds, words, or prayer, we tend to be happy. "Jesus went about doing good and curing all who had fallen into the power of the devil" (Acts 10:38, JB).

By simply uniting our sufferings to Christ and praying for others we have become pourers. The prayer of a sick, suffering person is very powerful and fruitful in itself. As mentioned before, when Venerable Archbishop Fulton J. Sheen visited a sick person, and asked that he or she offer a few minutes of their suffering for the intention of a talk he was going to give, he would receive power to be a great preacher through the prayers and suffering of the members of the Mystical Body of Jesus. The tree of the cross bears incalculable fruit.

Lord Jesus, please extend Your mercy toward us and make us the happy *pourers* You have called us to be. Thank You, Jesus. We trust in You.

HEALING THROUGH A SENSE OF HUMOR

"But Yahweh asked Abraham, 'Why did Sarah laugh and say "Am I really going to have a child now that I am old?" Is anything too wonderful for Yahweh? At the same time next year I shall visit you again and Sarah will have a son.' 'I did not laugh,' Sarah said, lying because she was afraid. But he replied, 'Oh yes, you did laugh'" (Genesis 18:13–15, JB).

I find this passage humorous, while at the same time conveying a serious and encouraging message. God kept His promise to Abraham and Sarah as He keeps all of His promises, and Sarah did give birth to Isaac when she was ninety years old and Abraham one hundred (see Genesis 17:17–18; 21:5). Truly, is anything too wonderful for God our Father? And we can be assured He is doing wonderful things in our lives at each and every step, in each and every circumstance. What seems impossible to us is not impossible for God. "For nothing is impossible to God" (Luke 1: 37, JB).

I think the best humor is that which we can relate to in our own lives and way of acting. Sarah, in her doubt (which God excused, since she went on to become a great matriarch), laughs at God's unfathomable promise. When God challenges her she denies having laughed; and God challenges her again to be honest. Can we not see ourselves in Sarah's reaction, both to doubt, and to be tempted to deny our culpability when caught? We are called to admit our weaknesses and exercise our free will in seeking the help we need from God, and in accepting the gifts He desires to pour out upon us.

I think most of us can benefit from an increased sense of humor, especially when it comes to ourselves. We need to admit the truth about ourselves as being needy, but beloved children of God, full of personal faults because we are human, but loved infinitely nonetheless. We need to accept this and to trust that our Merciful Father knows us perfectly, as He knew the complete truth about Sarah, and that He nonetheless unconditionally desires to pour out His seemingly impossible gifts upon each of us.

I often pray for an increased sense of humor in my life. Humor is a beautiful gift as long as it is not acquired at the detrimental expense of another; it is good have some laughs at the expense of oneself sometimes, which only help to increase the great and hard-won virtue of humility.

My main challenge toward living virtue all my life has been impatience. I believe God has a sense of humor. He may have thought something to the effect of, Okay, Jim, you are impatient. I will give you an arena in which to work on the virtue of patience. I have chosen you, and I will give you the great gift and responsibility of fourteen living children to raise. Love them and be patient with them as I am with you. Weakling that you are, you can do it with my help, which will not be lacking! "But he said to me, 'My grace is sufficient for you, for power is made perfect in weakness.' I will rather boast most gladly of my weaknesses, in order that the power of Christ may dwell with me" (2 Corinthians 12:9).

Okay, it's true, I'm a weakling. Admitting the truth about myself is liberating. Lord, help me; please grant me patience!

> Put on then, as God's chosen ones, holy and beloved, heartfelt compassion, kindness, humility, gentleness, and patience, bearing with one another and forgiving one

another, if one has a grievance against another; as the Lord
has forgiven you, so must you also do. And over all these
put on love, that is, the bond of perfection.

Colossians 3:12–14

When in my hospital room during the decisive hour of receiving
my stem-cell transplant, with the donor cells being infused into
my bloodstream, something came over me. By the grace of God,
I was in a very upbeat and humorous mood. There were a number
of people in the room for the occasion, including various medical
personnel and family members. It became a party atmosphere. I
began telling humorous stories to everyone present, and everyone
was smiling and laughing. I learned later that most people, when
receiving a stem-cell transplant, are very stiffly lying in bed, not
moving a muscle, and very apprehensive about the process.

I will tell you that I am not always this upbeat, but I believe
God gave me a special grace that day to be unafraid and joyful.
This helped everyone there, but most especially it helped me, as
the alternative would have been to suffer more due to my fear and
turning in on myself. God help me to have a good sense of humor
on a more consistent basis.

While hospitalized for twenty-eight days for the stem-cell
transplant, my family and I tried to make the best of things in a
positive way. We celebrated the birthdays of two of our children
in my hospital room during this time. A third was celebrated at
home with me participating by Skype. It was rather comical to
see numerous children of mine crammed into my room wearing
oversized surgical masks, gowns, and sterile gloves. Nonetheless it
was an upbeat party atmosphere.

Another time I ordered ice cream for my children, which they
greatly enjoyed as they looked out from the fifteenth-story window
of my hospital room mesmerized at how small the people and cars

were below. They began to look at visiting me in the hospital as an exciting adventure that was full of fun.

When my youngest two children, Shealagh, age five, and Brighde, age six, visited, I appealed to their imagination telling them about *Bridge to Terabithia* in the hospital hallway.[82] There was, in fact, a practice stairway consisting of three or four steps, leading to a landing facing a painting on the wall of a bridge depicting a forest and hills in the distance, hiding whatever might appeal to the imagination of children. I built up the excitement and enthusiasm to a fever pitch; we then visited this amazing *Bridge to Terabithia*. The stairs became the bridge while the painting represented the land which the bridge led to. They had a great time using their imagination. Since then, my children often refer back to this experience in a nostalgic way, both the younger children who participated and the older children who witnessed the experience.

On another occasion a few years ago, before my diagnosis, I was competing in a running race with several of my children at a park. As we were nearing the end of the race to culminate at a chain-link fence, which was as tall as me, I was winning. I decided that since this would likely be one of the last times I could win a race against my older children due to my getting older, I would run hard to the finish and bounce my shoulder off the fence to stop. Not a very smart idea!

Well, what I didn't know was that the chain-link fence was not attached to the horizontal pole at the top designed to support the fence like it was supposed to be, so when I went to bounce off of it, the fence gave way like the breeze. I ran virtually full speed into the pole. It was a tough pole, much tougher than my face. It hit significantly harder than any martial-arts opponent I had ever sparred with. The pole won. My forehead hit the pole, which of course did not give way at all, and I was knocked flat.

My children, who thought I was invincible, ran up laughing at Dad, the practical joker, and told me to stop kidding around, while I writhed on the ground in pain with blood pouring into my hat, which I had placed over my wounded eye. (I still proudly wear the hat, sanctified with my bloodstains.) This was yet another of numerous occasions where God saved me in spite of my foolhardiness.

As I was not a fan of going to the doctor, I taped the wound shut with some bandages. I was injured, but not down for the count. When we got home I wrote a sign, which we still have, saying: "Pain, I love it." I had my picture taken with it. I tried to have a sense of humor over the somewhat painful accident. I also wanted to teach my children a lesson.

Pain, I love it had been a favorite saying in my house, which I had started. I wanted to walk my talk. Not that pain in itself is good, but I wanted to thoroughly ingrain in my family the truth that pain is part of life, and that most everything worthy in life will involve some degree of pain, be it studying in school, or suffering an illness or cross, which will lead to an astounding good for me and others.

I am greatly inspired by the story of St. Lawrence, deacon and martyr. He was able to keep a sense of humor even during what had to have been excruciating suffering, as demonstrated in this brief account:

> In great anger, the Prefect condemned Lawrence to a slow, cruel death. The Saint was tied on top of an iron grill over a slow fire that roasted his flesh little by little, but Lawrence was burning with so much love of God that he almost did not feel the flames. In fact, God gave him so much strength and joy that he even joked. "Turn me over," he said to the judge. "I'm done on this side!" And just before he died, he said, "It's cooked enough now." Then he prayed that the city of Rome might be converted to Jesus and that the Catholic Faith might spread all over the world. After that, he went

to receive the martyr's reward. Saint Lawrence's feast day is August 10th.[83]

I believe that the ability to maintain a sense of humor amid such intense suffering is an extraordinary gift that can only be granted by God, but that He always stands ready to grant such a gift if we only humbly and confidently ask Him. We are weak. He is strong, and He always desires to share His strength with us.

I often turn to another saint, Thomas More, to ask his intercession with God that I be given a greater sense of humor. St. Thomas would pray for a sense of humor himself, which God graciously granted to him in abundance. God always answers our prayers in abundance. His prayer was: "Lord, give me a sense of humor and I will find happiness in life and profit for others."[84] Even in the moments leading up to his martyrdom for the truths of the Catholic faith on July 7, 1535, he was more concerned for others than for himself, in good humor, cracking jokes, and attempting to help others who had to fulfill or witness his execution to feel at ease. I am honored to have providentially been born on his Feast day, June 22.

> Early in the morning of July 7, Sir Thomas Pope, a friend, came to inform him that he was to die that day at nine o'clock. More thanked him, said he would pray for the king, and with talk of a joyful meeting in Heaven strove to cheer up his weeping friend. When the hour came he walked out to Tower Hill, and mounted the scaffold, with a jest for the lieutenant who helped him climb it.
>
> To the bystanders he spoke briefly, asking for their prayers and their witness that he died in faith of the Holy Catholic Church and as the king's loyal subject. He then knelt and repeated the psalm Miserere; after which he encouraged the executioner, though warning him that his neck was very short and he must take heed to "strike not

awry." So saying, he laid down his head and was beheaded at one stroke. His body was buried in the church of St. Peter-AD-Vincula within the Tower; his head, after being exposed on London Bridge, was given to Margaret and laid in the Roper vault in the church of St. Dunstan, outside the West Gate of Canterbury. There, presumably, it still is, beneath the floor under the organ, at the east end of the south aisle.[85]

Father, I know this is a selfish prayer as it will bring much happiness to me, but may we all be blessed with a good sense of humor and a cheerful disposition, at least the majority of the time, so that we can be a profit to others.

"May he grant us cheerful hearts" (Ecclesiasticus 50:25, JB).

HEALING THROUGH OUR MOTHER, MARY, LEADING TO THE WORD

"And Mary said:/ 'My soul proclaims the greatness of the Lord;/ my spirit rejoices in God my savior'" (Luke 1:46–47).

First, the reader should know that I am biased when it comes to the Blessed Virgin Mary. She is my great love. However, this great love does not diminish but only augments my love for others, such as my other great love, my wife Kathleen, and of course my own mother on earth. I have been totally consecrated to Mary for many years.

I am convinced that the Blessed Virgin Mary has been responsible for saving my life, both here on earth and eternally, on numerous occasions through her intercession with her Son, Jesus, who never denies any of her requests.

On one occasion in particular Mary saved me in a salient and unconcealed way. I am recalling a time about twelve years ago. There was a special Mass and a celebration afterward at my parish, St. Anthony, on the Feast of Our Lady of Guadalupe (one of the Blessed Virgin Mary's titles) in her honor. There was a major snowstorm that night. On the way home from the Mass and party on northbound Harlem Avenue, which has one lane in each direction approaching Route 30, there was a disabled vehicle blocking the northbound lane. I stopped behind it and decided to get out and lend assistance to the driver in front of us.

At some point I was standing next to our van near the driver's door, which I had exited. It was very loud with the wind and the noise of snowplows in the area. The windows of the van were up with Kathleen and the children inside the van. I looked north to the opposite, southbound lane and saw no vehicles traveling south, the way they were supposed to be traveling, and I turned to step out into that lane. As it turned out there was unexpectedly a vehicle passing my van northbound in the southbound lane from the direction that I did not expect. I was just about to step into the path of this vehicle, which as it turned out was traveling at a high rate of speed. At that precise moment I heard my name called gently but firmly, "Jim!" I stopped in my tracks before stepping out into the other lane. At that exact moment, I reacted to the warning and stopped. The vehicle passed at a high rate of speed, barely missing striking me. I would have stepped into its path and certainly been killed, had I not been warned.

At first I thought that my wife, Kathleen, had warned me, but she denied having done so. She had not seen the approaching vehicle. Besides, I could never have heard her because the windows were rolled up, and because of all of the exterior noise. I am convinced that it was the voice of Mary, Our Lady of Guadalupe, that saved my life in this extraordinary way.

There have been innumerable times that God, "author of saving acts" (Psalm 74:12, JB), has saved my life necessitated mostly from my own acts of stupidity, through the intercession of the Blessed Virgin Mary. After all, all graces that come to us pass through her. Think of it—what if Mary had said *no* to being the mother of Jesus? We would have all been lost in our sins. But her totally selfless response was: "I am the handmaid of the Lord," said Mary "...let what you have said be done to me" (Luke 1:38, JB).

Obviously God had some more trouble for me to stir up in the world, a plan for me, and a mission to fulfill; so He protected me, in spite of my appalling behavior.

I have often taken comfort and confidence in the following words of Our Lady of Guadalupe: "Listen, my son, to what I tell you now: do not be troubled nor disturbed by anything; do not fear illness nor any other distressing occurrence, nor pain. Am I not your mother? Am I not life and health? Have I not placed you on my lap and made you my responsibility? Do you need anything else?"[86]

Mary does everything well, but there is one apropos thing that she does especially well. That is she accompanies us at every moment in our suffering. When our Merciful Father has permitted us to hang and bleed on the cross, Mary, our Mother of the Sorrowful Heart, is always at the foot of our cross as she was at her Son's. "Near the cross of Jesus stood his mother" (John 19:25, JB). There is no one beside God who cares more about us than our Blessed Mother Mary. What unfathomable empathy she has for us! And there is no one who has more influence to intercede for us with Jesus than His own mother, Mary. And yes, she can and does intercede! Would we ever ask a friend to pray for us? Well, we can most certainly ask Mary to pray for us! She is as truly alive as you and I are, full of life and grace.

Mary is our mother as well. She is the *quintessential mother.* And it was God, Jesus Himself, who gave Mary to us as our mother when He said to John (who represented us all[87]): "This is your mother" (John 19:27, JB). We are called to make a place for Mary, our mother, in the home of our hearts. "And from that moment the disciple made a place for her in his home" (John 19:27, JB).

Mary's supreme empathy for each of us is similar to the empathy she experienced at the foot of the cross of her Son, Jesus. Because of her immaculate love and purity she suffered more empathetically and intensely than all the physical sufferings combined one could imagine. She felt the pain of a mystical sword, sharper and more penetrating than any steel sword, pierce her soul. This is the pain our Mother, Mary, takes on for us, because she loves us in the most authentic and efficacious way wherein her love is extraordinarily costly to her. "And a sword will pierce your own soul too…" (Luke 2:35, JB).

Mary is constant and faithful, no matter what, in praying and interceding for us. She is offering our pain and suffering to our Father in heaven, uniting it with the passion and death of her Son, Jesus, so that the bountiful fruit of love and everlasting life will result for our soul as well as others.

There is transferability to others of the merits won by our prayers and sufferings. This transferability applies toward the living here on earth as well as the souls in purgatory, who are all part of the Mystical Body of Christ. Expounding upon an analogy from Venerable Archbishop Fulton J. Sheen, one can compare this to healthy blood being transfused into the veins of a sick person.[88] That healthy blood will circulate through the entire body from the tip of the toes to the top of the head. The merits of our sacramental and prayer life united with our cross, pain, and suffering are transferred or transfused into the Mystical Body of Christ. These merits are applied in a true and mysterious way to particular individuals—but I dare say, to everyone. Since blood flows through the entire body nourishing every cell, there is not a single person living in the world or in purgatory who does not benefit in some way from our merits. We must keep in mind that these merits are not really thanks to us, but they are gifts and privileges of participation in the merits of Jesus, which our Heavenly Father of Mercies permits. "Now I rejoice in my sufferings for your sake, and in my flesh I am filling up what is lacking in the afflictions of Christ on behalf of his body, which is the church" (Colossians 1:24).

All of these prayers, sufferings, and merits pass through the Immaculate Heart of our Blessed Mother Mary. Those who do not believe that Mary is their mother may turn to John 19:25–27: "Standing by the cross of Jesus were his mother and his mother's sister, Mary the wife of Clopas, and Mary of Magdala." Note this representation of humanity, sinners and saints alike, including Mary of Magdela, a huge sinner who became an even greater saint, as can each of us. "When Jesus saw his mother and the disciple there whom he loved [John], he said to his mother, 'Woman, behold, your son.'" We see, from Jesus's own lips, that in one of His final words as He approached His death (keeping in mind the last words of the dying are always supremely important words) He proclaimed Mary as our mother. John represents each of us as sons of Mary, and as sons of the Church. What a gift! What a mother!

To those who don't believe that Mary is their mother, it is true that God gave us a free will; however, our free will does not change objective realities. If I were to disown my own human mother and claim that she was never my mother, I could claim that all I wanted, but she would still in truth be my mother. Mary is truly our mother. There are many who do not know or accept this, often through no fault of their own; however, this makes Mary no less their mother. For example, although an infant in the womb has never seen the face of his mother, and may not be able to comprehend the person of his mother (though I think he or she does so in an intuitive and profound way, as we also can comprehend our Mother, Mary, if we allow Jesus to heal us spiritually), this would make the mother no less existent. Not only that, the infant is constantly benefitting from the love, generosity, and nurturing of his mother, acknowledgment or not.

Our Mother, Mary, loves, protects and nurtures each of us at every moment whether we acknowledge it or not. The only element potentially lacking is our acknowledgment of and gratefulness toward our Mother, Mary. And should we ever ask the Blessed Virgin Mary to intercede for us in some way, we can be absolutely confident that she will, and that her Son, Jesus, will never refuse her anything for our good.

See, Mary is a giver, a pourer. In other words she is always giving and pouring herself out for others. She never has been and never will be centered on herself. This is one of the reasons why she is supremely happy, though in a mysterious way at the same time sorrowful because of her deep empathy toward each of us, beyond our imagination, with the suffering of her children. Like any good mother Mary feels the pain of her suffering children to a great extent—more than they do themselves. Every mother understands this. Multiply the sorrowful empathy of the most loving and sorrowful mother you know by the largest number you can think of, and multiply that by the same number a trillion times, and we have some very dim understanding of the Sorrowful and Immaculate Heart of Mary. By the grace of God I honor Mary with a rosary each day; my prayer is that the reader will accept the invitation to do the same. (See appendix.)

Some may claim that the rosary is a repetitive prayer that is not meaningful. Volumes can and have been written on the beauty and efficacy of the rosary, but to give an insight, which I again borrow from Venerable Archbishop Fulton J. Sheen, with every Hail Mary we are in a sense simply saying to Jesus and Mary, *I love you!*[89] Could we ever really say or hear "I love you" in a heartfelt way too often to or from someone we love?

Even those devoted to the Blessed Virgin Mary often underestimate her unfathomable love for us and her power of intercession. We are called to return that love. Just to say her name...*Mary*...with a deep love and tenderness while contemplating her and her virtues is enough in my very convinced opinion to assure the saving of one's soul. Not that we could go forward from that moment living our lives steeped in sin with no concern about repentance or the need of God's mercy; rather, because the utterance of her sublime name with love is enough to win so many tremendous graces from our Lord Jesus through Mary, one will naturally be propelled toward growth in a life of sanctity from that moment on.

As a matter of fact when we let the name…Mary…emanate from our heart and lips one can envision with certainty our Lord Jesus, seated at the right hand of our merciful Father, suddenly leaning forward with rapt attention to our soul, all our needs, all our prayers, and intentions. For when we love His Mother we have suddenly become part of His special inner circle upon which He constantly lavishes extraordinary gifts through His Holy Spirit, her Spouse. Blessed be the name of Mary, the Theotokos, the Mother of God!

Let's reflect on Genesis 24:15–27 (JB) wherein Abraham's servant had set out to choose a wife for his son Isaac. This event prefigures the Blessed Virgin Mary.

"He had not finished speaking when Rebekah came out. She was the daughter of Bethuel, son of Milcah, wife of Abraham's brother Nahor. She had a pitcher on her shoulder."

This pitcher would later contain water, representing the Holy Spirit in the living waters to be poured out upon us. The pitcher was filled representing the Blessed Virgin Mary who was and is full of grace. "Hail, full of grace" (Luke 1:28, Douay Rheims Bible). Grace is compared with water in John 7:37–39:

> On the last and greatest day of the feast, Jesus stood up and exclaimed, "Let anyone who thirsts come to me and drink. Whoever believes in me, as scripture says: 'Rivers of living water will flow from within him.'" He said this in reference to the Spirit that those who came to believe in him were to receive. There was, of course, no Spirit yet, because Jesus had not yet been glorified."

Returning to Genesis: 24:15–27 "The girl was very beautiful, and a virgin; no man had touched her." This describes the Blessed Virgin Mary very well. "But Mary said to the angel, 'How can this be, since I have no relations with a man?'" (Luke 1:34).

Returning to Genesis: 24:15–27 "She went down to the spring, filled her pitcher and came up again."

The spring represents the living waters which Jesus Christ gives us. "Running to meet her, the servant said, 'Please give me a little water to drink from your pitcher.'" Do we all not thirst for these living waters that make us righteous in God's eyes?

"She replied, 'Drink, my lord,' and she quickly lowered her pitcher on her arm and gave him a drink." Mary always *quickly* leads us to Christ to drink of His grace.

"When she had finished letting him drink, she said, 'I will draw water for your camels, too, until they have had enough.'" The Blessed Virgin Mary is the model of humility and service. She also sees to every need and detail of our lives, especially when we are consecrated to her.

"She quickly emptied her pitcher into the trough, and ran to the well again to draw water, and drew water for all the camels while the man watched in silence, wondering whether Yahweh had made his journey successful or not." The Blessed Virgin Mary has access to the well of the living waters of Jesus Christ, and liberally empties these upon us. Like this servant we can only contemplate the Blessed Virgin Mary and the graces she obtains for us in profound silence and wonder.

"When the camels had finished drinking, the man took a gold ring weighing half a shekel, and put it through her nostril, and put on her arms two bracelets weighing ten gold shekels, and he said, 'Whose daughter are you? Please tell me.'" This shows the royalty of our Blessed Lady. There are many among you who do not know the Blessed Virgin Mary and ask, "Whose daughter are you?" She desires very much for us to get to know her and come to her with veneration, and with all of our needs.

"'Is there room at your father's house for us to spend the night?' She answered, 'I am the daughter of Bethuel, the son whom Milcah bore to Nahor.' And she went on, 'We have plenty of straw and fodder, and room to lodge.'" The Blessed Virgin Mary constantly prays, works, and intercedes for us to enter our Father's house to lodge for all eternity.

"Then the man bowed down and worshipped Yahweh saying, 'Blessed be Yahweh, God of my master Abraham, for he has not stopped showing kindness and goodness to my master. Yahweh has guided my steps to the house of my master's brother.'" We see how the servant praises God and recognizes His providential action in his life and mission. Truly, through the intercession of the Blessed Virgin Mary, we are led to God where we discover His love and providential action for our good in every moment and circumstance of our lives, and we come to worship Him.

> Hail Mary, full of grace, the Lord is with thee, blessed art thou amongst women and blessed is the fruit of thy womb, Jesus. Holy Mary, mother of God, pray for us sinners now and at the hour of our death. Amen.

Jesus said to the woman at the well in John 4:10–14:

> "If you knew the gift of God and who is saying to you, 'Give me a drink,' you would have asked him and he would have given you living water." [The woman] said to him, "Sir, you do not even have a bucket and the cistern is deep; where then can you get this living water? Are you greater than our father Jacob, who gave us this cistern and drank from it himself with his children and his flocks?" Jesus answered and said to her, "Everyone who drinks this water will be thirsty again; but whoever drinks the water I shall give will never thirst; the water I shall give will become in him a spring of water welling up to eternal life."

May we all come to drink of the living spring of water of Jesus welling up to eternal life!

I will conclude with something I wrote by the grace of God on the gospel of John 1:1–5 on February 10, 2002, the eve of the Feast of Our Lady of Lourdes, which I pray will enkindle the fire of divine love in your heart. This is the fruit of contemplation, an expression of what this gospel passage means to me, and of how the Blessed Virgin Mary has interceded for me and how God has loved me and acted in my life. The contemplation does not describe experiences of the world that are seen, heard, smelled, and felt, and which happen in time and space. Rather, it describes things of the world of the unseen, of the Spirit—which are even more real and infinitely more beautiful than what we experience with our worldly senses, and which can only dimly be expressed in words, because there we encounter in a special way the infinite love of Love Himself. His name is Jesus!

> In the beginning was the Word,/ and the Word was with God,/ and the Word was God./ He was in the beginning with God./ All things came to be through him,/ and without him nothing came to be./ What came to be through him was life,/ and this life was the light of the human race;/ the light shines in the darkness,/ and the darkness has not overcome it.

John 1:1–5

What is this light that shines in the darkness? Dearest Father in heaven, You were in the beginning; I did not exist in the beginning, yet I did exist in Your thought, for You have always thought of me. Oh, generous Father in heaven, You had but one thought in all of eternity, and that thought is expressed in one Word, and that Word is Everything to You, and to me. That Word is Your only beloved Son.

Yet I was contained from all eternity in Your one thought expressed in Your one, most perfect Word, who says all there is or can be said—I, who have nothing good to offer but what You have given me. All I have been able to create on my own is sin, which killed me, though I thought I lived.

Deceived as I was, You spoke Your Word, who lived Your will and was crucified. By my ingratitude and sin, I became the lance that was driven into the Heart of Your Word, which You wrote on the wood of the Cross. Oh, what sublime surprise to find my sin absorbed in the blood of Your Son. This Heart has a light so infinitely pure and bright that the darkness of my sins is utterly and completely destroyed. Your Word's death has brought me to life. In Your Word's Heart a happy mystery has been revealed: my redemption has always been contained in Your one thought as expressed in Your one Word. I need only remain in the Heart of Your Word, where my littleness and total dependency on You will always be illuminated. There the darkness will never overcome me. But where do I find this Heart in the reality of the world, which You have made through Your Word? I will need to find Your Word and stay with Him.

Then she, my Mother, appeared on the scene most powerfully, yet at the same time gently hiding herself in the Light. It was she who gave her "yes" to give the Word His Sacred Heart of Flesh. She took my hand. I resisted, but saw that I should follow. She was inestimably stronger than me, and could have overcome me by force, but she nobly chose to permit my surrender.

I was starving, weak, blind, lame, leprous, and seemingly dead, but she had defended the flicker of life that had remained in me. I asked her to bend near to me that she might hear the faint whisper I could barely muster, and I said, "No matter what, please never let go of my hand. Arrange my life. I accept all that this entails. Only, I am weak, so keep me always under the protection of your mantle."

She led me toward the Heart of the Word. This is an infinitely magnanimous and merciful Heart. She led but preferred to hide herself in the brightness of the Light. She showed me the door to the Heart of the Word. The door was her own heart, which was Immaculate. As she helped me into her heart I experienced a piercing of sorrow. I was pierced by the same sword that was imbedded in Her heart. Although my flesh rebelled against this pain, I found it sweet and pleasant in my soul. I found a mysterious joy and peace mixed inexplicably with this sorrow. It was good. I remained in the door, this Mother's heart, which I discovered was not only a door, but an integral part contained within the Heart of the Word. I found my remedy, my life. My life is the Word.

This Word I realized was His Body, Blood, Soul, and Divinity, which He offered as Food. This is the Bread of Life. There was Blood and Water pouring upon me in this Heart of the Word. This Word which always contained me, breathed His Spirit upon me. I found this Spirit and this Word, both one with the Father, dwelling in my heart. What a beautiful and supreme mystery! All of our hearts were one. Our blood all ran together mixed as one in the Heart of the Word. I had found perfect happiness (though not yet fulfilled), but at the same time a consuming sorrow.

I looked for my Mother who stepped out of hiding, and I contemplated her immeasurable sorrow. The Spirit showed me this sorrow was contained in the Love of the Word, and that one cannot share His love without sharing His sorrow to some degree. The more one loves, the more one shares this sorrow; hence the immeasurable sorrow of my Mother. Her sorrow was being experienced for me and a multitude of other souls who had always been contained in the one thought of the Father, and His one Word.

My Mother brought me to the Word. He showed me a tiny place in His Heart where my own heart would fit like a completed puzzle, but I was free to choose whether to place my heart there or not. I saw that if I refused there would always be that empty place in the Heart of the Word. In order to place my heart there I was asked first by the Word if I would drink of His cup. As I took the cup, I saw it was the blood of the Word made flesh, and mingled with my own blood and sins, which had been consumed in His blood. As I drank I was filled with peace and joy, yet prevailing sorrow. This sorrow was as nothing compared to the sorrow of my Mother, yet it seemed more than I could bear. At this moment the Light revealed my total dependence on the Father, Word, and Spirit, and I threw myself into the abyss of their infinite mercy. I was filled with life from the Life, who touched and inflamed my heart with a fire that burned with a zeal to bring more souls to this Heart. I experienced in the Light that I was too weak to do anything at all, yet the Word gave me the Bread of Life, His Flesh.

I was filled with an invincible strength. My flesh seemed unchanged, so fragile and weak, yet the Spirit lifted me up with this strength. I needed to relieve the burning zeal in my heart infused with this invincible strength. It was impossible to contain. I would either spend it, or be devoured by it.

After being given this Life, I learned that I was to die to myself. Another sublime mystery—I must die to live. If I would die every moment and every day, I would live. I was given the unearned privilege of drinking of the cup of the Word, which meant being conformed to the Word, and dying like Him to live and to help others to live. Powerless, I found power by surrendering and tumbling into this abyss of mercy, even unto death.

I had no courage to die, so I gave my Mother permission to ask her Spouse, the Spirit, to strike me over and over with the sword in my Mother's heart. And He did. And He does. And He shall. Sometimes she hides so that the brightness of the Light will overcome the darkness, so I will remember who thought of me, and spoke of me, and loved me, even when I was yet dead in sin, not yet dying to myself with the Word, through Him and in Him.

And when the sword does not strike, there is an emptiness, for only in dying is there life. And I know that life is worth living, now that living means dying. And most of all I know that Mother knows best, and her hand is warm and firm, and I long for her whispers that are spoken in the wordless words of her Spouse, words of love, encouragement, and comfort, as well as words of correction.

My Heavenly Mother is always true and constant. I cannot see her with my eyes as I am immersed in her heart. Can an infant see his mother when wrapped in a mantle, and held against her heart? I am even closer as I listen from within to her beating heart, which is burning with a fire and zeal for souls greater than all other created hearts. There is room in this heart for the hearts of every soul that ever was or will be created.

Another beautiful mystery—this most humble and meek created heart has a capacity for all other hearts, because the Word wants this. And when a heart is in her heart it is secure in the Heart of the Word.

Can a heart choose to be in the Heart of the Word without being contained in the heart of our Mother? Yes, in the one sense of honoring the gift of free will; but in essence, no, since even these perplexed hearts are sharing the blood of the Mother's heart, whether conscious of this or not, and since the heart of the Mother is one with the Heart of the Word, the hearts of these souls are in essence one with the Mother's heart.

What of those who do not know of the Mother? How much does an infant in the womb know of his mother and her features and personality? Does this limitation make the infant any less a child of his mother, or any less loved and cared for by her? This love and care is not dependent on the knowledge or acceptance of the infant in the womb.

Oh, Mother of all mankind, pray for us now and at the hour of our death, amen! Pray for us every moment as we struggle to die to ourselves. Happy the man who is dying every hour of every day, to be conformed to the Word, through the help of his Mother, so when he dies he will live forever in perfect happiness and fulfillment in the presence of the Father, in the Heart of the Word, filled beyond understanding with the Holy Spirit, all one. Thanks be to God, Almighty yet All merciful.

EPILOGUE

Grace to you and peace from God our Father and the Lord Jesus Christ. I give thanks to my God always on your account for the grace of God bestowed on you in Christ Jesus, that in him you were enriched in every way, with all discourse and all knowledge, as the testimony to Christ was confirmed among you, so that you are not lacking in any spiritual gift as you wait for the revelation of our Lord Jesus Christ. He will keep you firm to the end, irreproachable on the day of our Lord Jesus [Christ]. God is faithful, and by him you were called to fellowship with his Son, Jesus Christ our Lord.

1 Corinthians 1:3–9

Thanks be to God as of July 2, 2012 my health is exceptional. I am cancer free and living full and joyfully without any physical restrictions. As a matter of fact I walked and jogged a 5K race with my family just two days ago. After learning my place in the race I was consoled by Jesus's words, "Thus the last will be first, and the first, last" (Matthew 20:16, JB). But what a joy to just participate!

November 1, 2011 Praise the Lord! Today is All Saints Day. I went to see my stem cell doctor and learned that based on a recent bone marrow test I am totally cancer free.

If I remain cancer free at the three year mark following the bone marrow transplant date I will be considered cured completely. We still have to deal with graft versus host disease, which he added a medication for, but as always I leave everything in the merciful hands of Jesus, the Blessed Virgin Mary, and all the holy Saints and Angels. I was also told that 98% of the cells in the bone marrow are now from the donor, which is as good as it gets. Therefore, the results of the bone marrow transplant are as perfect as they can be. This is in spite of the fact that I went into the bone marrow transplant with a significant percentage of leukemia cells in the bone marrow. Ideally one enters into a bone marrow transplant with very little or no cancer present, in other words in a strong remission. Therefore, it is remarkable, and in my opinion a miracle that the bone marrow transplant was so successful in eradicating the cancer for me. But regardless, it is always God's merciful hand working behind all forms of healing whether seemingly natural or supernatural.

I do want to profoundly thank and credit Venerable Archbishop Fulton J. Sheen as the primary intercessor in heaven through the Immaculate Heart of the Blessed Virgin Mary to Jesus for my healing, as I and many others prayed to him for my healing from the beginning of my illness. He is at work in heaven helping us, even more so than when he lived his remarkably fruitful life on earth.

I prayed prayers of thanksgiving with my family. I also went in the evening to visit Jesus in the Adoration Chapel to give Him thanks for my healing. I wanted to be like the man in the gospel who came back to thank Him when Jesus asked where the other nine were who were healed. "Jesus said in reply, 'Ten were cleansed, were they not? Where are the other nine? Has none but this foreigner returned to give thanks to God?' Then he said to him, 'Stand up and go; your faith has saved you'" (Luke 17:17–19).

I am also incredibly grateful to all the many who have prayed so incessantly for me and my family. I owe them more than I can express.

If God is extending my life on earth through a physical healing does it mean that I am more favored or loved than another who does not receive this same gift? By no means! Our merciful Father is simply unfolding His perfect, infinitely loving, and unique plan for each of us for our highest good. He deserves our unconditional trust.

My story continues. We know that its ending will be in accord with the perfect and good will of God, so it will have the best possible conclusion, as will your story.

Anything good and helpful in this book is from the Holy Spirit. Anything poorly done or prideful is from me, and I am sure there is much. I have tried to write what I believe God wanted me to write. I hope the reader comes away with some helpful insights, encouragement, increased hope, faith, and fortitude, as well as some useful resolutions. I am sure the Holy Spirit has something singular and profound to say to each individual reader.

What I have tried to convey is that Jesus is the One who heals in every conceivable way, and I have tried to tell about His incredible love, goodness, and mercy. He is "Faithful and True" (Revelation 19:12, JB). Will my cancer remain gone indefinitely? Will the reader or his or her loved one be physically healed from cancer or some other serious illness, or be delivered from some adversity? I do not know. But what I do know is that Jesus, our Lord, is with us. He is "always loving, always loyal" (Psalm 86:16, JB). He is interested in and in command of every detail of our individual lives. Nothing can ever happen outside of His will. We are secure in Him. He is bringing an astounding good out of everything we encounter. He loves us infinitely. Whatever the outcome, it will truly be for the best.

Jesus is the *Divine Physician*. He is the One who heals in diverse and mysterious ways that are often beyond our human comprehension. I pray that you, as a suffering soul (and that includes everyone), have received at least some faint insight into a few of the ways God has been at work in your mind, body, soul, and spirit for the good. Yes, much of the good He is accomplishing remains hidden until He greets us in eternity. God's ways are not our ways. He is a God of hidden ways. "Truly with you God is hidden, the God of Israel,/ the savior!" (Isaiah 45:15). He leads us along mysterious and hidden paths, always for our good.

I hope you, the reader, have received some consolation and encouragement. Perhaps you will accept and implement some of the means of healing and redemption referred to in this book. I hope you will see with greater clarity how our Most High and Merciful God has been working astonishing *healings* in your life in the various ways written about in this book as well as in others ways (and they are many) that the Holy Spirit may have revealed to you.

I would be remiss if I did not share with you, my special, eternal friends, the readers, the most precious gift and healing I have ever received, that of my membership in the Catholic Church. This gift is not imposed. Your freedom is absolutely respected, and I would always defend it to the best of my ability. It is a gift offered, out of love. The Catholic Church is the Mystical Body of Jesus Christ; its visible head is the Holy Father, the Pope. Its invisible Head is Jesus Christ. The Holy Spirit pours Himself out upon the Church, permeates, leads, and gives life to the Church, both as a whole and individually in each of its members.

If you believe you may be called to the fullness of faith in the Catholic Church, I encourage you to contact your local parish to inquire. Why did Jesus establish His Church? For the good of you, the reader, as if you were the only person ever created. The Church does not act outside of Christ. Everything the Church binds on earth is bound in heaven, and everything loosed on earth in loosed in heaven. "Amen, I say to you, whatever you bind on earth shall be bound in heaven, and whatever you loose on earth shall be loosed in heaven" (Matthew 18:18). Jesus has given this power and privilege of applying His incredible mercy to His Church out of love for us. His Church is supremely merciful. No sin or number of sins is unforgivable. How could they be greater than the infinite ocean of God's mercy? There is nothing God ever does that is not out of infinite LOVE.

The Church is the means by which the precious blood of Christ is poured out upon us for the remission of our sins. In fact, "without the shedding of blood there is no forgiveness" (Hebrews 9:22). And this blood is truly the most *precious healing balm* we can ever encounter. It is so precious that it will sooth us for all eternity.

I have not met most of you, but God knows who you are. I will never fail to remember you in my prayers and to thank God for each of you (see Ephesians 1:16–17). May I call you my friend, my brother, my sister? I offer my little share of the cross for each of you and your intentions. Count on these little prayers and offerings. May I ask for yours? If God should permit my life to end soon here on earth as a result of my cancer or some other reason, know for certain that I will be praying more fervently and effectively in heaven for each of you than if He had prolonged my life and mission on earth. Sinner that I am, I cannot imagine ending up anywhere else than heaven, because I love Jesus, and I trust completely in His infinite mercy. "It is all God's work" (2 Corinthians 5:17–18, JB). Thank You, Jesus.

I wish to borrow words from my great mentor, Venerable Archbishop Fulton J. Sheen, and to make those words my own to you, the reader.

The reason I want to go the heaven is because I want to be with love. Oh there will be surprises there, many of them.

First of all, there will be many people there whom we never expected to see there. There will also be a number of people absent who we thought would be there. Finally there will be one great surprise, the greatest of all, that you and I are there. I'll see you in heaven.[90]

This is my deepest prayer made in complete confidence in the mercy of Jesus. *The mountain has been cast into the sea!* (see Mark 11:22–25).

Yes, I pray we will all meet one day in heaven where we will have all eternity to reminisce about the beautiful and mysterious ways God has lovingly worked for the good in our lives. We will have everything in heaven, where we will be perfectly happy for all eternity. There is only one thing we will have nostalgia for which we cannot have in heaven (if nostalgia be possible in heaven, in the sense that it adds to our complete happiness). It is the gift that our infinitely wise God has given to each of us that was so amazingly efficacious in our healing and purification—our share of the cross, not the least of which was our difficult illnesses and adversities. We will understand then what a truly sublime gift the cross was, how we were healed through it, and how so many others benefited from our cross. May our Merciful God bless each of you and yours. May we meet again! In the Name of the Father, and of the Son, and of the Holy Spirit. Amen. I believe!

The writing of this book was completed on October 18, 2011, the Feast of St. Luke, Evangelist; also the eve of the Memorial of Isaac Jogues and John De Brébeuf, Priests and Martyrs, and Companions, Martyrs, also the eve of the two-year anniversary of my diagnosis. Praise the Lord!

QUALIFICATION

I wish to make the statement that I made every effort to assure that everything written in this book is in agreement with the teachings of the Catholic Church, including seeking the editorial review and advice of many holy theologians, Catholic Christian leaders, and the United States Conference of Catholic Bishops. Should there yet be anything written contradicting the truth of the Church's teachings, I would like to be made aware so that I might rectify the situation to the extent within my power and apologize. I have not been able to cover even a small portion of the beautiful truths the Church offers. That would be an impossible endeavor for me. Besides, for that purpose the quintessential and brilliant resource, the *Catechism of the Catholic Church*, already exists. I have tried to focus, more than anything else, on the infinite mercy of God. This is so fundamental that without this greatest attribute of God there would be really no point to anything, including the Church. In that case I would have no choice but to join the way of nihilism. Fortunately, we can be absolutely convinced that the mercy of Jesus does exist and is available for each of us.

Though this book is directed toward persons of any and all religions and beliefs, I can never betray my love for the Catholic Church, which is synonymous with my love for Jesus, my Lord and merciful Savior.

HEALING
SCRIPTURE PASSAGES

One can return to the following Scripture passages in daily prayer for inspiration, hope, and fortitude along with the countless movements of the Holy Spirit which He has in store for anyone who prays, especially when using Scripture. The selected passages only skim the surface of the blessings to be found in the Bible. There are incalculable additional gems beside these for each individual, salted throughout Scripture, containing new, unique insights and consolations that can never be exhausted.

Or a man is chastened on his bed by pain/ and unceasing suffering within his frame,/ So that to his appetite food becomes repulsive,/ and his senses reject the choicest nourishment./ His flesh is wasted so that it cannot be seen,/ and his bones, once invisible, appear;/ His soul draws near to the pit,/ his life to the place of the dead.

If then there be for him an angel,/ one out of a thousand, a mediator,/ To show him what is right for him/ and bring the man back to justice,/ He will take pity on him and say,/ "Deliver him from going down to the pit;/ I have found him a ransom."/ Then his flesh shall become soft as a boy's;/ he shall be again as in the days of his youth./ He shall pray and God will favor him;/ he shall see God's face with rejoicing./ He shall sing before men and say,/ "I sinned and did wrong,/ yet he has not punished me accordingly./ He delivered my soul from passing to the pit,/ and I behold the light of life."

Lo, all these things God does,/ twice, or thrice, for a man,/ Bringing back his soul from the pit/ to the light, in the land of the living.

Job 33:19–30

Happy is the man whom God reproves!/ The Almighty's chastening do not reject./ For he wounds, but he binds up;/ he smites, but his hands give healing.

Job 5:17–18

And I said to you: do not take fright, do not be afraid of them, Yahweh your God goes in front of you and will be fighting on your side as you saw him fight for you in Egypt. In the wilderness, too, you saw him: how Yahweh carried you, as a man carries his child, all alone the road you traveled on the way to this place.

Deuteronomy 1:29–33, JB

You are blessed for having made me glad. What I feared has not happened; instead you have treated us with mercy beyond all measure.

Tobit 8:16, JB

I keep Yahweh before me always, for with him at my right hand nothing can shake me.

Psalm 16:8, JB

They assailed me on my day of disaster, but Yahweh was my support; he freed me, set me at large, he rescued me, since he loves me.

Psalm 18:18–19, JB

Now I know that Yahweh saves his anointed, and answers him from his holy heaven with mighty victories from his own right hand.

Psalm 20:6, JB

Yahweh is my shepherd, I lack nothing.

Psalm 23:1, JB

Yahweh is my strength, my shield, my heart puts its trust in him; I have been helped, my flesh has bloomed again. I thank him with all my heart.

Psalm 28:7, JB

You are a hiding place for me, you guard me when in trouble, you surround me with songs of deliverance.

Psalm 32:7, JB

Our soul awaits Yahweh, he is our help and shield; our hearts rejoice in him, we trust in his holy name. Yahweh, let your love rest on us as our hope has rested in you.

Psalm 33:20–22, JB

They cry for help and Yahweh hears and rescues them from all their troubles; Yahweh is near to the broken-hearted, he helps those whose spirit is crushed. Hardships in plenty beset the virtuous man, but Yahweh rescues him from them all; taking care of every bone. Yahweh will not let one be broken.

Psalm 34:17–20, JB

Then my soul will rejoice in Yahweh, exult that he has saved me. All my bones will exclaim, "Yahweh, who can compare with you in rescuing the poor man from the stronger, the needy from the man who exploits him?"

Psalm 35:9–10, JB

My helper, my saviour, my God, come and do not delay!

Psalm 40:17, JB

Whoever makes thanksgiving his sacrifice honours me; to the upright man I will show how God can save.

Psalm 50:23, JB

I, for myself, appeal to God and Yahweh saves me.

Psalm 55:16, JB

Unload your burden on to Yahweh, and he will support you; he will never permit the virtuous to falter.

Psalm 55:22, JB

Rest in God alone, my soul! He is the source of my hope; with him alone for my rock, my safety, my fortress, I can never fall; rest in God, my safety, my glory, the rock of my strength. In God I find shelter; rely on him, people, at all times; unburden your hearts to him, God is a shelter for us.

Psalm 62:5–8, JB

For my part, I pray to you, Yahweh, at the time you wish; in your great love, answer me, God, faithful in saving power.

Psalm 69:13, JB

I promise that, ever hopeful, I will praise you more and more, my lips shall proclaim your righteousness and power to save, all day long.

Psalm 71:14–15, JB

Now that I am old and grey, God, do not desert me; let me live to tell the rising generation about your strength and power, about your heavenly righteousness, God. You have done great things; who, God, is comparable to you? You have sent me misery and hardship, but you will give me life again, you will pull me up again from the depths of the earth, prolong my old age, and once more comfort me.

Psalm 71:18–21, JB

I rescue all who cling to me, I protect whoever knows my name, I answer everyone who invokes me, I am with them when they are in trouble; I bring them safety and honour. I give them life, long and full, and show them how I can save.

Psalm 91:14–16, JB

Then they called to Yahweh in their trouble and he rescued them from their sufferings, reducing the storm to a whisper until the waves grew quiet, bringing them, glad at the calm, safe to the port they were bound for.

Psalm 107:28–30, JB

Yahweh is righteous and merciful, our God is tenderhearted;
Yahweh defends the simple, he saved me when I was
brought to my knees.

Psalm 116:5–6, JB

No, I shall not die, I shall live to recite the deeds of
Yahweh; though Yahweh has punished me often, he has
not abandoned me to Death.

Psalm 118:17–18, JB

Support me as you have promised, and I shall live, do not
disappoint me of my hope. Uphold me, and I shall be safe.

Psalm 119:116–117, JB

Though I live surrounded by trouble, you keep me alive–to
my enemies' fury! You stretch your hand out and save me,
your right hand will do everything for me.

Psalm 138:7–8, JB

For every way, LORD! you magnified and glorified your
people;/ unfailing, you stood by them in every time and
circumstance.

Wisdom 19:22

Sheltered by your hand, the whole nation passed across, gazing at these amazing miracles. They were like horses at pasture, they skipped like lambs, singing your praises, Lord, their deliverer.

Wisdom 19:8–9, JB

Trust him and he will uphold you.

Ecclesiasticus 2:6, JB

Often I was in danger of death,/ but by these attainments I was saved./ Lively is the courage of those who fear the Lord,/ for they put their hope in their savior;/ He who fears the Lord is never alarmed, never afraid; for the Lord is his hope./ Happy the soul that fears the Lord!/ In whom does he trust, and who is his support?/ The eyes of the Lord are upon those who love him;/ he is their mighty shield and strong support,/ A shelter from the heat, a shade from the noonday sun,/ a guard against stumbling, a help against falling./ He buoys up the spirits, brings a sparkle to the eyes,/ gives health and life and blessing.

Sirach 34:12–17

I was at the point of death,/ my soul was nearing the depths of the nether world;/ I turned every way, but there was no one to help me,/ I looked for one to sustain me, but could find no one./ But then I remembered the mercies of the Lord,/ his kindness through ages past;/ For he saves those who take refuge in him,/ and rescues them from every evil./ So I raised my voice from the very earth,/ from the gates of the nether world, my cry./ I called out: O Lord, you are my father,/ you are my champion and my savior;/ Do not abandon me in time of trouble,/ in the midst of storms and dangers./ I will ever praise your name/ and be constant in my prayers to you./ Thereupon the LORD heard my voice,/ he listened to my appeal;/ He saved me from evil of every kind/ and preserved me in time of trouble./ For this reason I thank him and I praise him;/ I bless the name of the LORD.

Sirach 51:6–12

They will turn to Yahweh who will listen to them and heal them.

Isaiah 19:22–23, JB

But Yahweh is waiting to be gracious to you, to rise and take pity on you, for Yahweh is a just God; happy are all who hope in Him.

Isaiah 30:18, JB

But those who hope in Yahweh renew their strength, they put out wings like eagles. They run and do not grow weary, walk and never tire.

Isaiah 40:31, JB

I have chosen you, not rejected you, do not be afraid, for I am with you; stop being anxious and watchful, for I am your God. I give you strength, I bring you help, I uphold you with my victorious right hand.

Isaiah 41:9–10, JB

For I, Yahweh, your God, I am holding you by the right hand; I tell you, "Do not be afraid, I will help you."

Isaiah 41:13, JB

Listen to me, faint hearts, who feel far from victory. I bring my victory near, already it is close, my salvation will not be late.

Isaiah 46:12–13, JB

Strengthen the hands that are feeble,/ make firm the knees that are weak,/ Say to those whose hearts are frightened:/ Be strong, fear not!/ Here is your God,/ he comes with vindication;/ With divine recompense/ he comes to save you.

Isaiah 35:3–4

Go, tell Hezekiah: Thus says the LORD, the God of your father David: I have heard your prayer and seen your tears.

I will heal you: in three days you shall go up to the LORD's temple; I will add fifteen years to your life.

Isaiah 38:5

Do not be afraid.

Isaiah 54:4, JB

For the mountains may depart, the hills be shaken, but my love for you will never leave you.

Isaiah 54:10, JB

I am with you to save you and to deliver you—it is Yahweh who speaks.

Jeremiah 15:20, JB

But look, I will hasten their recover and their cure; I will cure them and let them know peace and security in full measure.

Jeremiah 33:6–7, JB

I will rescue you that day—it is Yahweh who speaks-and you will not be delivered into the hands of the men you fear. I will see that you escape: you are not going to fall to the sword; you will escape with your life, because you have put your trust in me- it is Yahweh who speaks.

Jeremiah 39:17–18, JB

Take courage, my children, call on God: he who brought disaster on you will remember you. As by your will you first strayed away from God, so now turn back and search for him ten times as hard; for as he brought down those disasters on you, so will he rescue you and give you eternal joy.

Baruch 4:27–29, JB

So as he stepped ashore he saw a large crowd; and he took pity on them and healed their sick.

Matthew 14:13–14, JB

During the fourth watch of the night, he came toward them, walking on the sea. When the disciples saw him walking on the sea they were terrified. "It is a ghost," they said, and they cried out in fear. At once [Jesus] spoke to them, "Take courage, it is I; do not be afraid." Peter said to him in reply, "Lord, if it is you, command me to come to you on the water." He said, "Come." Peter got out of the boat and began to walk on the water toward Jesus. But when he saw how [strong] the wind was he became frightened; and, beginning to sink, he cried out, "Lord, save me!" Immediately Jesus stretched out his hand and caught him, and said to him, "O you of little faith, why did you doubt?" After they got into the boat, the wind died down. Those who were in the boat did him homage, saying, "Truly, you are the Son of God."

Matthew 14:25–33

And if you have faith, everything you ask for in prayer you will receive.

Matthew 21:22, JB

And know that I am with you always; yes, to the end of time.

Matthew 28:20, JB

Do not be afraid; only have faith.

Mark 5:37, JB

Everything is possible for anyone who has faith.

Mark 9:24, JB

Let the little children come to me; do not stop them; for it is to such as these that the kingdom of God belongs.

Mark 10:14–15, JB

Amen, I say to you, whoever says to this mountain, "Be lifted up and thrown into the sea," and does not doubt in his heart but believes that what he says will happen, it shall be done for him. Therefore I tell you, all that you ask for in prayer, believe that you will receive it and it shall be yours. When you stand to pray, forgive anyone against whom you have a grievance, so that your heavenly Father may in turn forgive you your transgressions.

Mark 11:23–25

There is no need to be afraid, little flock, for it has pleased your Father to give you the kingdom.

Luke 12:32, JB

This sickness will end not in death, but in God's glory, and through it the son of God will be glorified.

John 11:4, JB

I have told you all this so that you may find peace in me. In the world you will have trouble, but be brave: I have conquered the world.

John 16:33, JB

We do not want you to be unaware, brothers, of the affliction that came to us in the province of Asia; we were utterly weighed down beyond our strength, so that we despaired even of life. Indeed, we had accepted within ourselves the sentence of death, that we might trust not in ourselves but in God who raises the dead. He rescued us from such great danger of death, and he will continue to rescue us; in him we have put our hope [that] he will also rescue us again, as you help us with prayer, so that thanks may be given by many on our behalf for the gift granted us through the prayers of many.

2 Corinthians 1:8–11

You will have in you the strength, based on his own glorious power, never to give in, but to bear anything joyfully, thanking the Father, who has made it possible for you to join the saints and with them to inherit the light.

Colossians 1:11–12, JB

God has called you and he will not fail you.

1 Thessalonians 5:24, JB

Be as confident now, then, since the reward is so great. You will need endurance to do God's will and gain what he has promised.

Hebrews 10:35–36, JB

You will have to suffer only for a little while: the God of all grace who called you to eternal glory in Christ will see that

317

all is well again: he will confirm, strengthen, and support you. His power lasts forever and ever. Amen.

1 Peter 5:10–11, JB

Think of the love that the Father has lavished on us, by letting us be called God's children; and that is what we are.

1 John 3:1, JB

Do not be afraid; it is I, the First and the Last; I am the Living One...

Revelation 1:17–18, JB

APPENDIX

I like to think of the Ten Commandments as the "Ten Rules of Love and Happiness." After all, we were given them by God for our good.

> And now, Israel, what does the LORD, your God, ask of you but to fear the LORD, your God, and follow his ways exactly, to love and serve the LORD, your God, with all your heart and all your soul, to keep the commandments and statutes of the LORD which I enjoin on you today for your own good?
>
> Deuteronomy 10:12–13

Confession Guide for Adults[91]

EXAMINATION OF CONSCIENCE

1. I am the Lord your God. You shall not have strange gods before me.
   -Do I give God time every day in prayer?
   -Do I seek to love Him with my whole heart?

-Have I been involved with superstitious practices, or have I been involved with the occult?

-Do I seek to surrender myself to God's word as taught by the Church?

-Have I ever received Communion in the state of mortal sin?

-Have I ever deliberately told a lie in confession, or have I withheld a mortal sin from the priest in confession?

-Are there other "gods" in my life? Money, Security, Power, People, etc.?

2. You shall not take the name of the Lord your God in vain.
    -Have I used God's name in vain—lightly or carelessly?
    -Have I been angry with God?
    -Have I wished evil upon any other person?
    -Have I insulted a sacred person or abused a sacred object?

3. Remember to keep holy the Lord's Day.
    -Have I deliberately missed Mass on Sundays or Holy Days of Obligation?
    -Have I tried to observe Sunday as a family day and a day of rest?
    -Do I do needless work on Sunday?

4. Honor your father and your mother.
    -Do I honor and obey my parents?
    -Have I neglected my duties to my spouse and children?
    -Have I given my family good religious example?
    -Do I try to bring peace into my home life?
    -Do I care for my aged and infirm relatives?

5. You shall not kill.
    -Have I had an abortion or encouraged or helped anyone to have an abortion?

-Have I physically harmed anyone?

-Have I abused alcohol or drugs?

-Did I give scandal to anyone, thereby leading him or her into sin?

-Have I been angry or resentful?

-Have I harbored hatred in my heart?

-Have I mutilated myself through any form of sterilization?

-Have I encouraged or condoned sterilization?

-Have I engaged, in any way, in sins against human life such as artificial insemination or in vitro fertilization?

-Have I participated in or approved of euthanasia?

6. You shall not commit adultery.

-Have I been faithful to my marriage vows in thought and action?

-Have I engaged in any sexual activity outside of marriage?

-Have I used any method of contraception or artificial birth control in my marriage?

-Has each sexual act in my marriage been open to the transmission of new life?

-Have I been guilty of masturbation?

-Do I seek to control my thoughts and imagination?

-Have I respected all members of the opposite sex, or have I thought of other people as mere objects?

-Have I been guilty of any homosexual activity?

-Do I seek to be chaste in my thoughts, words, and actions?

-Am I careful to dress modestly?

7. You shall not steal.

-Have I stolen what is not mine?

-Have I returned or made restitution for what I have stolen?

-Do I waste time at work, school, and home?

-Do I gamble excessively, thereby denying my family of their needs?

-Do I pay my debts promptly?

-Do I seek to share what I have with the poor?

-Have I cheated anyone out of what is justly theirs, for example, creditors, insurance companies, big corporations?

8. You shall not bear false witness against your neighbor.

-Have I lied?

-Have I gossiped?

-Do I speak badly of others behind their back?

-Am I sincere in my dealings with others?

-Am I critical, negative, or uncharitable in my thoughts of others?

-Do I keep secret what should be kept confidential?

-Have I injured the reputation of others by slanders?

9. You shall not desire your neighbor's wife.

-Have I consented to impure thoughts?

-Have I caused them by impure reading, movies, television, conversation, or curiosity?

-Do I pray at once to banish impure thoughts and temptations?

-Have I behaved in an inappropriate way with members of the opposite sex: flirting, being superficial, etc.?

10. You shall not desire your neighbor's goods.

-Am I jealous of what other people have?

-Do I envy the families or possessions of others?

-Am I greedy or selfish?

-Are material possessions the purpose of my life?

A GUIDE TO CONFESSION

How to go to Confession

1. You always have the option to go to confession anonymously, that is, behind a screen, or you can go face-to-face, if you so desire.

2. After the priest greets you in the name of Christ, make the Sign of the Cross. He may choose to recite a reading from Scripture, after which you say: "Bless me, Father, for I have sinned. It has been (state how long) since my last confession. These are my sins."

3. Tell your sins simply and honestly to the priest. You might even want to discuss the circumstances and the root causes of your sins and ask the priest for advice or direction.

4. Listen to the advice the priest gives you and accept the penance from him. Then make an Act of Contrition for your sins.

5. The priest will then dismiss you with the words of praise: "Give thanks to the Lord for He is good." You respond: "For His mercy endures forever." The priest will then conclude with: "The Lord has freed you from your sins. Go in peace." And you respond by saying: "Thanks be to God."

6. Spend some time with our Lord thanking and praising Him for the gift of His mercy. Try to perform your penance as soon as possible.

PRAYER BEFORE CONFESSION

O most merciful God! Prostrate at your feet, I implore your forgiveness. I sincerely desire to leave all my evil ways and to confess my sins with all sincerity to you and to your priest. I am a sinner; have mercy on me, O Lord. Give me a lively faith and a firm hope in the Passion of my Redeemer. Give me, for your mercy's sake, a sorrow for having offended so good a God. Mary, my Mother, refuge of sinners, pray for me that I may make a good confession. Amen.

AN ACT OF CONTRITION

Oh my God,
I am sorry for my sins with all my heart.
In choosing to do wrong
and failing to do good,
I have sinned against you,
whom I should love above all things.
I firmly intend, with your help,
to do penance,
to sin no more,
and to avoid whatever leads me to sin.
Our Savior Jesus Christ
suffered and died for us.
In His name, my God, have mercy. Amen.

HOW TO PRAY THE ROSARY[92]

The Rosary is a Scripture-based prayer. It begins with the *Apostles' Creed*, which summarizes the great mysteries of the Catholic faith. The *Our Father*, which introduces each mystery, is from the gospels. The first part of the *Hail Mary* is the angel's words announcing Christ's birth and Elizabeth's greeting to Mary. St. Pius V officially added the second part of the *Hail Mary*. The Mysteries of the Rosary center on the events of Christ's life. There are four sets of Mysteries: Joyful, Sorrowful, Glorious, and—added by Pope John II in 2002—the Luminous.

The repetition in the Rosary is meant to lead one into restful and contemplative prayer related to each Mystery. The gentle repetition of the words helps us to enter into the silence of our hearts, where Christ's spirit dwells. The Rosary can be said privately or with a group.

The Five Joyful Mysteries are traditionally prayed on the Mondays, Saturdays, and Sundays of Advent:

1. The Annunciation
2. The Visitation
3. The Nativity
4. The Presentation in the Temple
5. The Finding in the Temple

The Five Sorrowful Mysteries are traditionally prayed on the Tuesday, Friday, and Sundays of Lent:

1. The Agony in the Garden
2. The Scourging at the Pillar
3. The Crowning with Thorns
4. The Carrying of the Cross
5. The Crucifixion and Death

The Five Glorious Mysteries are traditionally prayed on the Wednesday and Sundays outside of Lent and Advent:

1. The Resurrection
2. The Ascension
3. The Descent of the Holy Spirit
4. The Assumption
5. The Coronation of Mary

The Five Luminous Mysteries are traditionally prayed on Thursdays:

1. The Baptism of Christ in the Jordan
2. The Wedding Feast at Cana
3. Jesus's Proclamation of the Coming of the Kingdom of God
4. The Transfiguration
5. The Institution of the Eucharist

PRAYERS OF THE ROSARY

The Apostles' Creed
I believe in God, the Father almighty creator of heaven and earth.
I believe in Jesus Christ, his only Son, Our Lord.
He was conceived by the power of the Holy Spirit
and born of the Virgin Mary.
He suffered under Pontius Pilate,
was crucified, died, and was buried.
He descended to the dead.
On the third day he rose again.
He ascended into heaven,

and is seated at the right hand of the Father.
He will come again to judge the living and the dead.

I believe in the Holy Spirit,
the holy catholic Church,
the communion of saints,
the forgiveness of sins,
and the resurrection of the body,
and the life everlasting.
Amen.

The Our Father
Our Father, who art in heaven,
hallowed be thy name;
thy kingdom come;
thy will be done on earth as it is in heaven.
Give us this day our daily bread;
and forgive us our trespasses
as we forgive those who trespass
against us;
and lead us not into temptation,
but deliver us from evil.
Amen.

The Hail Mary
Hail Mary, full of grace,
the Lord is with you!
Blessed are you among women,
and blessed is the fruit of your womb, Jesus.
Holy Mary, Mother of God,
pray for us sinners,
now and at the hour of our death.
Amen.

The Glory Be (The Doxology)
Glory be to the Father, the Son, and the Holy Spirit.
As it was in the beginning is now and ever shall be
world without end.
Amen.

The Hail Holy Queen (The Salve Regina)
Hail, holy Queen, mother of mercy,
hail, our life, our sweetness, and our hope.
To you we cry, the children of Eve;
to you we send up our sighs,
mourning and weeping in this land of exile.
Turn, then, most gracious advocate,
your eyes of mercy toward us;
lead us home at last
and show us the blessed fruit of your womb,
Jesus:
O clement, O loving, O sweet Virgin Mary.

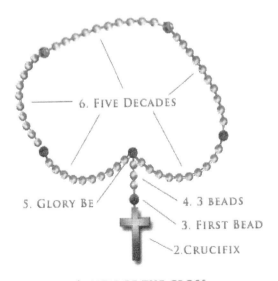

6. FIVE DECADES

5. GLORY BE

4. 3 BEADS

3. FIRST BEAD

2. CRUCIFIX

1. SIGN OF THE CROSS

PRAYING THE ROSARY

Familiarize yourself and/or your group with the prayers of the rosary.

Make the Sign of the Cross.

Holding the Crucifix, say the *Apostles' Creed.*

On the first bead, say an *Our Father.*

Say three *Hail Marys* on each of the next three beads.

Say the *Glory Be.*

For each of the five decades, announce the Mystery, then say the *Our Father.*

While fingering each of the ten beads of the decade, next say ten *Hail Marys* while meditating on the Mystery. Then say a *Glory Be.* (After finishing each decade, some say the following prayer requested by the Blessed Virgin Mary at Fatima: "O my Jesus, forgive us our sins, save us from the fires of hell, lead all souls to Heaven, especially those who have most need of your mercy.")

After saying the five decades, say the "Hail, Holy Queen", followed by this dialogue and prayer:

V. Pray for us, O holy Mother of God.

R. That we may be made worthy of the promises of Christ.

Let us pray: O God, whose only-begotten Son, by his life, death, and resurrection,

has purchased for us the rewards of eternal life,

grant, we beseech thee, that while meditating on these mysteries of the most holy Rosary,

of the Blessed Virgin Mary,

we may imitate what they contain

and obtain what they promise,

through the same *Christ our Lord.*

Amen.

ABOUT THE AUTHOR

James Littleton, speaker, life coach, spiritual guide, cancer sojourner, media guest; co-author, with his wife Kathleen, of *Better by the Dozen, Plus Two: Anecdotes and a Philosophy of Life from a Family of Sixteen.* Jim and his wife, Kathleen are parents of nineteen children, fourteen living on earth, ages twenty-six to six, and five living in heaven. He is available as a speaker, coach, or retreat or workshop presenter on a wide range of Healing, Faith and Family topics. He has had numerous guest appearances on television and radio including EWTN, and has been featured in articles in numerous publications including Zenit and the Chicago Tribune. James can be reached with questions, comments, interview or speaking engagement requests at jamesmlittleton@gmail.com.

ENDNOTES

1   Read more about Michael Novak at http://www.michaelnovak.net/index.cfm?fuseaction=Home.welcome

2   See Fulton J. Sheen, *State of the Church*, cassette tape, St Joseph Communications.

3   *Catechism references*: OP 46: formula of absolution

4   See Fulton J. Sheen, *Treasure in Clay: The Autobiography of Fulton J. Sheen* (San Francisco: Ignatius Press, 1993), 129–31.

5   *Catechism of the Catholic Church* (Citta del Vaticano: Libreria Editrice Vaticana, 1994), http://www.vatican.va/archive/ENG0015/_INDEX.HTM.

6   See Fulton J. Sheen, *Through the Year with Fulton Sheen*, comp. and ed. Henry Dietrich (San Francisco: Ignatius Press, 2003), 140.

7   Saint John of the Cross, *The Collected Works of Saint John of the Cross*, trans. Kieran Kavanaugh, O.C.D., and Otilio Rodriguez, O.C.D. (Washington, DC: ICS Publications, 1991), 74.

8   *The Liturgy of the Hours*, International Commission on English in the Liturgy, 1975 (New York: Catholic Book Publishing Corp., 1975).

9   *DIARY, Saint Maria Faustina Kowalska: Divine Mercy in My Soul* © 1987 Congregation of the Marians of the Immaculate Conception, Stockbridge, MA 01263. All Rights Reserved. Used with permission.

10 Blessed Columba Marmion, *Union with God: Letters of Spiritual Direction by Blessed Columba Marmion*, selected and annotated by Dom Raymond Thibaut. trans. Mother Mary St. Thomas (Bethesda, MD: Zaccheus Press, 2006), 119.

11 Luis M. Martinez, D.D., *Only Jesus*, trans. Sister Mary St. Daniel, B.V.M. (St. Louis, MO: B. Herder Book Co., 1962), 168.

12 *Catechism* references: cf. *Rite of Baptism of Children* 62.

13 Read further: *Catechism* 1596

14 *Catechism* references: Revelation 1:6; cf. Revelation 5:9–10; 1 Peter 2:5,9.

15 *Catechism* references: *Lumen Gentium* 10 § 1.

16 *DIARY, Saint Maria Faustina Kowalska: Divine Mercy in My Soul* © 1987 Congregation of the Marians of the Immaculate Conception, Stockbridge, MA 01263. All Rights Reserved. Used with permission.

17 Fulton J. Sheen, *Through the Year with Fulton Sheen*, comp. and ed. Henry Dietrich (San Francisco: Ignatius Press, 2003), 225.

18 Luis M. Martinez, D.D., *Only Jesus*, trans. Sister Mary St. Daniel, B.V.M. (St. Louis, MO: B. Herder Book Co., 1962), 157.

19 http://www.hebrew4christians.com/Glossary/glossary.html

20 Wiki Info, "Mount Zion," http://www.wikinfo.org/English/index.php/Mount_Zion.

21 *Catechism* references: cf. Ephesians 3:14.

22 *Catechism* references: Matthew 19:6; cf. Genesis 2:24;

23 *Catechism* references: *Familiaris consortio* 19.

24 "Memorial of SS. Isaac Jogues and John de Brébeuf," *The Liturgy of the Hours*, International Commission on English in the Liturgy, 1975 (New York: Catholic Book Publishing Corp., 1975).

25 See Fulton J. Sheen, *Through the Year with Fulton Sheen*, comp. and ed. Henry Dietrich (San Francisco: Ignatius Press, 2003), 225.

26 See Fulton J. Sheen, *Treasure in Clay: The Autobiography of Fulton J. Sheen* (San Francisco: Ignatius Press, 1993), 129.

27 See Fulton J. Sheen, *Through the Year with Fulton Sheen*, comp. and ed. Henry Dietrich (San Francisco: Ignatius Press, 2003), 179.

28 See Fulton J. Sheen, exact source not found.

29   See Fulton J. Sheen, *Holy Ambassadors*, cassette tape, St Joseph Communications, side two.

30   See Fulton J. Sheen, *Through the Year with Fulton Sheen*, comp. and ed. Henry Dietrich (San Francisco: Ignatius Press, 2003), 70.

31   *Catechism* references: 2 Peter 1:4.

32   *Catechism* references: St. Irenaeus, *Adv. haeres.* 3, 19, 1: PG 7/1, 939.

33   *Catechism* references: St. Athanasius, *De inc.* 54, 3: PG 25, 192B.

34   *Catechism* references: St. Thomas Aquinas, *Opusc.* 57, 1–4.

35   http://en.wikipedia.org/wiki/Cyrene,_Libya

36   *DIARY, Saint Maria Faustina Kowalska: Divine Mercy in My Soul*© 1987 Congregation of the Marians of the Immaculate Conception, Stockbridge, MA 01263. All Rights Reserved. Used with permission.

37   See Fulton J. Sheen, *Meaning of Suffering*, cassette tape, St. Joseph Communications.

38   *Catechism* references: 1 Corinthians 2:11.

39   *Catechism* references: John 16:13.

40   *Catechism* references: John 14:17.

41   *Catechism references: Cf. Rom 8:29; Council of Trent (1547): DS 1609–1619.*

42   Read further about what experts say at *http://www.prolife. com/BIRTHCNT.html*

43   *Catechism* references: *Familiaris consortio* 30.

44   *Catechism* references: *Humanae vitae* 11.

45   *Catechism* references: *Humanae vitae* 12; cf. Pius XI, encyclical, *Casti connubii.*

46   *Catechism* references: *Humanae vitae* 16.

47   *Catechism* references: *Humanae vitae* 14.

48   *Catechism* references: *Familiaris consortio* 32.

49   This is one of the links: http://www.sciencedaily.com/ releases/2007/02/070221065200.htm

50   Cardinal Nguyen Van Thuan, *Testimony of Hope: Spiritual Exercises of John Paul II*, trans. Julia Mary Darrenkamp and Anne Eileen Heffernan (Boston: Pauline Books & Media, 2000).

51   James M. Littleton, written in Eucharistic adoration chapel, February 1999, revised July 21, 2011.

52   See Fulton J. Sheen, exact source not found.

53   *Catechism* references: *Ordo paenitantiae* 46: formula of absolution.

54 *DIARY, Saint Maria Faustina Kowalska: Divine Mercy in My Soul* © 1987 Congregation of the Marians of the Immaculate Conception, Stockbridge, MA 01263. All Rights Reserved. Used with permission.

55 *Catechism* references: Matthew 12:31; cf. Mark 3:29, Luke 12:10.

56 *Catechism* references: cf. Blessed John Paul II, *Dominum et Vivificanum* 46.

57 Reverend Hugo Hoever, S.O. Cist., Ph.D., *Lives of the Saints for Every Day of the Year* (New York: Catholic Book Publishing Company, 1993)., 381

58 Reverend Hugo Hoever, S.O. Cist., Ph.D., *Lives of the Saints for Every Day of the Year* (New York: Catholic Book Publishing Company, 1993), 254–55.

59 We see in the above passage how Jesus continues to work through the Holy Spirit through His Church, with Peter as the first Pope, and the other apostles as the first bishops.

60 See Fulton J. Sheen, *Through the Year with Fulton Sheen*, comp. and ed. Henry Dietrich (San Francisco: Ignatius Press, 2003), 60.

61 *Catechism* references: cf. Hebrews 7:25–27.

62 *Catechism* references: *Lumen gentium* 3; cf. 1 Corinthians 5:7.

63 *Catechism* references: Luke 22:19–20.

64 *Catechism* references: Matthew 26:28.

65   *Catechism* references: Council of Trent (1562): Denzinger-Schonmetzer, *Enchiridion Symbolorum, definitionum et declarationum de rebus fidei et morum* (1965) 1740; cf. 1 Corinthians 11:23; Hebrews 7:24, 27.

66   *Catechism* references: Council of Trent (1562) *Doctrina de ss. Missae sacrificio*, c. 2: Denzinger-Schonmetzer, *Enchiridion Symbolorum, definitionum et declarationum de rebus fidei et morum* (1965) 1743; cf. Hebrews 9:14, 27.

67   *Catechism* references: *Lumen gentium* 11.

68   *Catechism* references: *Presbyterorum ordinis* 5.

69   See Fulton J. Sheen, *The Greatest Novena Ever Preached! About the Simplest Life Ever Lived...St. Therese the Little Flower on the Occasion of the 100ᵗʰ Anniversary of Her Birth, Given at the Carmelite Church, Whitefriar Street, Dublin, 1973*, cassette tape, talk 4.

70   See Servant of God Archbishop Luis Martinez, exact source not found.

71   Easter Vigil, *Roman Missal, Third Edition*, International Commission on English in the Liturgy, 2010 (Woodridge, IL: Midwest Theological Forum, 2011), 472.

72   Fulton J. Sheen, *The Meaning of Suffering*, cassette tape, St Joseph Communications, side one.

73   *Catechism* references: John 5:29; cf. Daniel 12:2.

74   *Catechism* references: Luke 24:39.

75   *Catechism* references: Lateran Council IV (1215): Denzinger-Schonmetzer, *Enchiridion Symbolorum, definitionum et declarationum de rebus fidei et morum* (1965) 801; Philippians 3:21; 1 Corinthians 15:44.

76   *Catechism* references: 1 Corinthians 15:35–37,42,52,53.

77   *Catechism* references: St. Irenaeus, *Adv. haeres.* 4,18,4–5:PG 7/1,1028–1029.

78   *Catechism* references: 1 Corinthians 6:13–15,19–20.

79   See Catholic-Pages.com, "St. Maximilian Kolbe," 2007, http://www.catholic-pages.com/saints/st_maximilian.asp.

80   See Fulton J. Sheen, *The Greatest Novena Ever Preached! About the Simplest Life Ever Lived…St. Therese the Little Flower on the Occasion of the 100ᵗʰ Anniversary of Her Birth, Given at the Carmelite Church, Whitefriar Street, Dublin, 1973*, cassette tape, talk 9.

81   Fulton J. Sheen, *Through the Year with Fulton Sheen*, comp. and ed. Henry Dietrich (San Francisco: Ignatius Press, 2003), 189–90.

82   Referring to the bridge in the 2007 Disney/Walden Media feature film *Bridge to Terabithia*

83   Catholic Online, "St. Lawrence – Martyr," http://www.catholic.org/saints/saint.php?saint_id=366.

84   Saint Thomas More holy card, Bridge Building Images, Inc.

85   "Saint Thomas More, Martyr, Chancellor of England," Eternal Word Television Network (taken from *Lives of Saints*, published by John J. Crawley & Co., Inc.), http://www.ewtn. com/library/mary/thomasmo.htm.

86   Words of Our Lady of Guadalupe to St. Juan Diego in 1531: "Our Lady of Guadalupe," Angelfire, http://www.angelfire. com/ri/prayers4life/guadalupe.html.

87   A partial theological explanation to this claim is that Jesus called Mary, His mother, *Woman*, referring back to Genesis 3:14-15, which made it clear He was referring to the new Eve, mother of us all, as was the first Eve. You can read further for some helpful information at http://www. thecatholictreasurechest.com/eve.htm

88   See Fulton Sheen, *Holy Ambassadors*, cassette tape, St Joseph Communications, side two.

89   See Fulton J. Sheen, *Your Life is Worth Living*, 331.

90   Fulton Sheen, *Through the Year with Fulton Sheen*, 2250.

91   "Confession Guide for Adults," *National Catholic Register*, EWTN News, Inc., 2011, http://www.ncregister.com/info/ confession_guide_for_adults

92   "How to Pray the Rosary," United States Conference of Catholic Bishops, 2011, http://usccb.org/prayer-and-worship/devotionals/rosaries/how-to-pray-the-rosary.cfm.

BIBLIOGRAPHY

Catechism of the Catholic Church. Citta del Vaticano: Libreria Editrice Vaticana, 1994. http://www.vatican.va/archive/ENG0015/_INDEX.HTM.

Catholic Online. "St. Lawrence – Martyr." http://www.catholic.org/saints/saint.php?saint_id=366.

Catholic-Pages.com. "St. Maximilian Kolbe." 2007. http://www.catholic-pages.com/saints/st_maximilian.asp.

"Confession Guide for Adults." *National Catholic Register.* EWTN News, Inc., 2011. http://www.ncregister.com/info/confession_guide_for_adults.

Easter Vigil. *Roman Missal, Third Edition.* International Commission on English in the Liturgy, 2010. Woodridge, IL: Midwest Theological Forum, 2011.

The Holy Bible Douay-Rheims Version. With revisions and footnotes (in the text in italics) by Bishop Richard Challoner, 1749–52. Taken from a hardcopy of the 1899 Edition by the John Murphy Company. The Latin Vulgate (Biblia Sacra Vulgata) Clementine Version. Translation from Greek and other languages into Latin by Saint Jerome, about 382 A.D. http://www.drbo.org/chapter/49001.htm.

Hoever, Reverend Hugo, S.O. Cist., Ph.D. *Lives of the Saints for Every Day of the Year.* New York: Catholic Book Publishing Company, 1993.

"How to Pray the Rosary." United States Conference of Catholic Bishops, 2011, http://usccb.org/prayer-and-worship/devotionals/rosaries/how-to-pray-the-rosary.cfm.

The Jerusalem Bible Reader's Edition, New York: Doubleday, 1966.

John of the Cross, Saint. *The Collected Works of Saint John of the Cross.* Translated by Kieran Kavanaugh, O.C.D., and Otilio Rodriguez, O.C.D. Washington, DC: ICS Publications, 1991.

DIARY, Saint Maria Faustina Kowalska: Divine Mercy in My Soul © 1987 Congregation of the Marians of the Immaculate Conception, Stockbridge, MA 01263. All Rights Reserved. Used with permission.

Lectionary for Mass for Use in the Dioceses of the United States of America, second *typical edition*. Washington, DC: Confraternity of Christian Doctrine, Inc.: © 2001, 1998, 1997, 1986, 1970.

Liturgy of the Hours, The. International Commission on English in the Liturgy, 1975. New York: Catholic Book Publishing Corp., 1975.

Marmion, Blessed Columba. *Union with God: Letters of Spiritual Direction by Blessed Columba Marmion.* Selected and

Annotated by Dom Raymond Thibaut. Translated by Mother Mary St. Thomas. Bethesda, MD: Zaccheus Press, 2006.

Martinez, Luis M., D.D. *Only Jesus.* Translated by Sister Mary St. Daniel, B.V.M. St. Louis, MO: B. Herder Book Co., 1962.

New American Bible with Revised New Testament and Revised Psalms. Washington, DC: Confraternity of Christian Doctrine, 1991.

"Our Lady of Guadalupe." Angelfire. http://www.angelfire.com/ri/prayers4life/guadalupe.html.

Saint Thomas More holy card. Bridge Building Images, Inc.

"Saint Thomas More, Martyr, Chancellor of England." Eternal Word Television Network. Taken from *Lives of Saints,* published by John J. Crawley & Co., Inc. http://www.ewtn.com/library/mary/thomasmo.htm.

Sheen, Fulton J. *The Greatest Novena Ever Preached! About the Simplest Life Ever* Lived…St. Therese the Little Flower on the Occasion of the 100th Anniversary of *Her Birth, Given at the Carmelite Church, Whitefriar Street, Dublin, 1973.* Cassette tape.

Sheen, Fulton J. *Holy Ambassadors.* Cassette tape. St. Joseph Communications.

Sheen, Fulton J. *The Meaning of Suffering.* Cassette tape. St. Joseph Communications.

Sheen, Fulton J. *State of the Church.* Cassette tape. St. Joseph Communications.

Sheen, Fulton J. *Through the Year with Fulton Sheen*. Compiled and edited by Henry Dietrich. San Francisco: Ignatius Press, 2003.

Sheen, Fulton J. *Treasure in Clay: The Autobiography of Fulton J. Sheen*. San Francisco: Ignatius Press, 1993.

Sheen, Fulton J. *Your Life is Worth Living: The Christian Philosophy of Life*. Schnecksville, PA: St. Andrew's Press, 2001.

Wiki Info. "Mount Zion." http://www.wikinfo.org/English/index.php/Mount Zion.

Van Thuan, Cardinal Nguyen. *Testimony of Hope: Spiritual Exercises of John Paul II*. Translated by Julia Mary Darrenkamp and Anne Eileen Heffernan. Boston: Pauline Books & Media, 2000.